T0171604

Itching, sneezing, runny nose . . .

For the forty million Americans who suffer from allergic rhinitis (hay fever) because of airborne allergens, is there any hope of relief? Dr. Gillian Shepherd, a noted allergy expert, offers sufferers a guide to understanding, diagnosing, treating, and preventing these allergy symptoms, including:

- how and why you are affected by allergens
- strategies to avoid symptoms
- why you need to take the right medications at the right time
- how your doctor can help
- how to live a happy life with allergies— but without symptoms.

WHAT'S IN THE AIR?

The Complete Guide to Seasonal and
Year-Round Airborne Allergies

GILLIAN SHEPHERD, M.D., and
MARIAN BETANCOURT

POCKET BOOKS
New York   London   Toronto   Sydney   Singapore

The sale of this book without its cover is unauthorized. If you purchased this book without a cover, you should be aware that it was reported to the publisher as "unsold and destroyed." Neither the authors nor the publisher have received payment for the sale of this "stripped book."

The ideas, procedures, and suggestions in this book are not intended as a substitute for the medical advice of your trained health professional. All matters regarding your health require medical supervision. Consult your physician before adopting the suggestions in this book, as well as about any condition that may require diagnosis or medical attention. The authors and publisher disclaim any liability arising directly or indirectly from the use of the book.

An *Original* Publication of POCKET BOOKS

 POCKET BOOKS, a division of Simon & Schuster, Inc.
1230 Avenue of the Americas, New York, NY 10020

Copyright © 2002 by Gillian Shepherd, M.D. and Marian Betancourt

Grateful acknowledgment is made to The Task Force on Allergic Disorders, *The Allergy Report, 2000,* on which the illustrations in this book are based, with permission from the American Academy of Allergy, Asthma and Immunology.

All rights reserved, including the right to reproduce this book or portions thereof in any form whatsoever. For information address Pocket Books, 1230 Avenue of the Americas, New York, NY 10020

ISBN 978-1-4516-4639-9

First Pocket Books printing September 2002

10 9 8 7 6 5 4 3 2 1

For information regarding special discounts for bulk purchases, please contact Simon & Schuster Special Sales at 1-800-456-6798 or business@simonandschuster.com

Book design by Helene Berinsky
Front cover photo by John Millar/Stone

Printed in the U.S.A.

to my allergy patients who have taught me so much

—G.S.

to my family, past, present, and future, all linked by our IgE molecules

—M.B.

CONTENTS

PART II

How Your Doctor Can Help You

PART III

The Allergic Person's Survival Guide

WHAT'S IN
THE AIR?

INTRODUCTION

The Allergy Boom and the Hygiene Hypothesis

Not everyone is programmed to develop allergies. You have to inherit the tendency. If you have close family with a history of hay fever, asthma, hives, eczema, or specific food or drug allergies, there is a chance you will develop allergy symptoms.

When I was twelve, I baby-sat at a home where there was a cat. Until that time I had very limited exposure to cats, so I happily played with it. After a short time my eyes started to itch, so I rubbed them. Before I knew it, both my eyes were swollen and I could barely see. This was my introduction to allergies.

At that time I lived in Rochester, Minnesota. My family had moved there from Belfast, Northern Ireland, when I was ten. Shortly after the baby-sitting incident, I started to develop sneezing and a runny and stuffy nose in the late summer. The Mayo Clinic scratched my back with multiple substances and told me I was allergic to ragweed—"the king" of the pollens in the Midwest from August 15 to the first frost. There was no ragweed in the United Kingdom and it took me two seasons in Minnesota to develop the allergy. I had lots of company sneezing and sniffling away every September.

The main treatment then was Chlor-Trimeton, an antihistamine that made me snooze through my classes, so generally I just suffered with my tissue box at hand. My parents then told me that they had had allergy-related problems in the past. My father had hives as a child and my mother had asthma as a teenager. They both "outgrew" their allergies. Meanwhile, I was sneezing and itching and my brother was blissfully unaffected. Why me?

Just because my father had hives as a child and my mother had asthma as a teenager did not mean I was programmed to get these specific allergy problems. Instead, I inherited a tendency to get any one of the various types of allergies. In my case, this turned out to be nasal and eye symptoms from cats and ragweed pollen.

Your immune system is like your body's homeland defense system. It guards you against foreign invaders such as bacteria or cancer cells. Occasionally it mistakes itself for a foreign invader, reacting against part of your body. This causes autoimmune disease. In the case of allergy, the immune system overreacts to innocent substances such as cats or pollen particles in the air. Normal, nonallergic people don't overreact to these substances. But if you are allergic you end up with sneezing, runny or stuffy nose, and teary eyes.

The human immune system is a giant network. Think of it as a road map showing different routes. Some paths protect us from foreign substances such as infection and cancer. One of the main routes, however, leads to allergies. If you are programmed to be allergic, inhale a speck of dog allergen and your immune system will crank out quantities of a chemical called immunoglobin E (IgE). The IgE charges through your bloodstream and sticks to special cells in the lining of your nose, throat, and lungs. It then acts as a sentry. If it encounters dog allergen again, it tells the cell to pump out powerful chemicals such as histamine. These chemicals make your nose and eyes run and cause itching and inflammation, among other symptoms.

The same reaction can happen in the lining of the eyes, causing itching and swelling. In the lungs it causes asthma. If the allergy is severe and the allergy substance is inside the body (food, medicine, or a bee sting), the reaction can occur throughout the body resulting in hives or a life-threatening reaction called anaphylaxis, which can result in airway swelling and difficulty breathing. IgE, the "allergic antibody," is normally present in very low levels, but is found in larger quantities in people with allergies.

Allergies also wax and wane. A childhood allergy to inhaled substances often goes away, but others may later appear. In my case, I lost my allergy to ragweed but later developed one to tree pollen. Unfortunately, two of my three children also inherited this problem. My husband has no allergies, so it came from me.

My own experience with allergies contributed to my ultimate choice of medical specialty, although there was never a doubt that I would be involved in medicine. I grew up surrounded by doctors—my father and his two brothers, my brother, and most of my cousins practice medicine. There are eleven doctors in my immediate family. Nevertheless, my initial interest after college was a Ph.D. research program rather than medical school. I eventually became involved in immunology research and decided I needed a broader background and so finally switched to medical school.

During training in internal medicine I selected allergy immunology as a subspecialty because I was intrigued by the complexity of the immune system. Then and even more so now, immunology was the hot field. Most of the other subspecialties were based on an organ, such as the heart, or lungs. The immune system interacted with every part of the body. Even in the early days of research, it was evident that it was a very powerful system with a role in every other system in the body. As a victim of dysfunction of the immune system, it was clear to me that the answer to allergies lay in further understanding and then manipulating the immune system.

Today allergies are booming. And unlike the stock market this trend has been rising steadily. More than 60 million Americans—20 percent of the population—suffer from allergies and that number is fast increasing. According to the National Institutes of Health (NIH), 40 million people—the largest percentage of the allergic public in the United States—are coping with allergic rhinitis, commonly known as hay fever, and allergic conjunctivitis. This is probably a low estimate because allergies are often underreported. Allergies are now the sixth leading cause of chronic disease in the United States.

Medical scientists are not exactly sure why the incidence of allergies is increasing. The prevailing theory is that the current population—in the United States and other developed countries—has been brought up in an environment that is too clean. When the immune system has no infections to fight, it finds something else to pick on, like a grain of pollen or mold spores. This theory is called the hygiene hypothesis. It seems to be a problem of advanced countries, because in developing countries like India and China, allergies are less of a problem.

In the twentieth century, we wiped out many infectious diseases with improved sanitation and drinking water, and with the use of antibiotics. From the 1930s to the 1950s, Dr. Spock advised parents to keep babies away from other children to prevent the spread of germs. This may have been bad advice; we know now that if you are an only child you may be more likely to have allergies than children from a large family. Children who attend day-care centers seem to have fewer allergies, too, possibly because their immune systems are actively engaged in fighting off infections. If this explanation for increasing allergies is true—that is, that we are exposed to fewer infections so our immune system defaults to allergy production—then we may be making the situation worse by exposing our children to more indoor allergy substances. Our children stay inside more, watching TV and computer screens instead of playing outside. This exposes them to indoor allergens such as pets, dust mites, and cockroaches.

A study in Scandinavia showed that the prevalence of allergic rhinitis increased from 4.4 percent to 8.4 percent between 1971 and 1981. In England, Scotland, and Wales, allergic rhinitis was found to occur in 12 percent of all children born during one week in 1958, but in 23.3 percent of those born during one week in 1970.

We are on the forefront of many new treatments as a result of advances in molecular biology, enabling us to manipulate the immune and allergy system by redirecting it back to fighting infections. If we succeed, allergies will be less prevalent. An anti-IgE drug is in the last stages of testing necessary before FDA approval. This drug may also have a potent role in the field of food and drug allergy. Many other substances are being investigated in an attempt to decrease the system's tendency to overreact. We can't "cure" the problem yet, because we can't reprogram the genetic system, but we hope to eventually be able to manipulate it to decrease the amount of allergies.

In the meantime, there is a great deal you can do. The goal of an allergist is to help you manage your allergies so that they do not interfere with the enjoyment of life. That's the reason for this book. By teaching you what is in the air and how it travels, you can learn to avoid some of the worst allergy situations. By helping you understand how to manage the air in your home, you can make it as allergy proof as possible. And also, by outlining the techniques and dynamics of medical therapy, we hope to help you use medications and work with your doctor in a way that will keep allergies under control.

We are focusing here on allergic rhinitis (hay fever) and allergic conjunctivitis, because these problems affect the largest number of people, but we hope this book will give you a greater understanding of all allergy-related conditions. There are chapters about coping with allergens on the job, helping your children with allergies, and where to go to get away from your allergies. Like any chronic illness, dealing with allergies takes a combination of understanding, self-management, prevention, and medication.

—Gillian Shepherd, M.D.

PART I

An Allergy Primer

1

WHY YOU ARE ALLERGIC

If you have allergies, you might say you have a slightly schizophrenic immune system. When you inhale an airborne allergen, such as pollen or mold, your immune system sees a foreign invader and it rushes into action to protect you. Such protective action is great against harmful bacteria, but in the case of an allergen, like cat or pollen, the system is making much ado about nothing dangerous. As a result, you sneeze, get a runny nose, teary eyes, or worse. You may have inherited this "altered reaction" (the definition of allergy) in your immune system, but you won't truly become allergic unless you are sensitized to an allergen. In other words, you need to be exposed to large doses of an allergen—or allergens—over time to become allergic.

Defining Allergens

An allergen is any foreign substance capable of inducing the immune system reaction that produces allergy symptoms. This results in too much IgE antibody inside your body. Common allergens include airborne proteins, pollen, mold spores, and various foods and drugs. Scientists also call these allergens "antigens."

Every season gives us something to sneeze at. Tree pollens in the spring, grasses in the summer, and ragweed floating through those brisk fall breezes, keep us sneezing. And we haven't even mentioned mold, dust mites, and pets, the source of big year-round allergens inside the home.

Some allergen terms are misleading, by the way. You may think you are allergic to cat or dog dander. Dander is the flaked-off skin of the animal and it is not an allergen. The allergen is in the animal's secretions that are attached to the dander or the fur. A cat licks its fur, then, as the cat walks about, tiny dried flakes of saliva break off, and the allergen in that saliva goes into the air. So that we don't perpetuate the misleading term *dander*, throughout the book we'll call it what it is: animal allergen or protein.

Unfortunately, lots of other things are blowing in the wind, too, such as increasing air pollution from industry and automobiles. While diesel fumes, ozone, and other pollutants are not allergens per se, they irritate our airways and make us more sensitive to allergens.

For allergens to become airborne and capable of being inhaled, they have to be tiny—1 to 5 microns. This means they are a millionth of a meter, or many times smaller than the dot at the end of this sentence. They also have to have certain chemical characteristics, and we'll get to that.

THE MAIN INHALED ALLERGENS

There are six primary airborne allergens you inhale.

- Pollens
- Molds
- Dust mite fecal droppings
- Animal protein
- Cockroach fecal droppings
- Latex particles

There are some other allergens, but these are the ones to which most of us are allergic.

Your respiratory tract is a perfect port of entry for allergens, and breathing them in may affect your *entire* respiratory tract from nose to lungs. Ragweed pollen, for example, breathed in through the nose of someone sensitive to it, causes allergic rhinitis, or if it reaches the lungs, may cause an asthma attack.

Animal allergens can also provoke asthma as well as allergic rhinitis.

But this doesn't happen until you have an allergy—or allergies. Let's see how that develops.

Remember the conditions that set you up for allergies.

1. You are genetically programmed.

2. You are exposed to allergens several times to stimulate the immune system to make too much IgE antibody.

The Genetic Setup

A family history of allergy is the single most important factor predisposing a child to develop diseases such as allergic rhinitis and asthma. The inherited tendency is called "atopy," and it increases the likelihood of developing allergic disease following exposure to allergens. Studies conducted over the last 30 years show the estimated risk of allergy to be 50 percent if one parent has a history of allergy and 66 percent if both parents have it.

THE IGE MOLECULE

IgE antibodies attach themselves to mast cells in tissue and basophils in the blood. These cells are produced in your bone marrow. Basophils are white blood cells that congregate around the invading molecules. Mast cells are found in connective tissue throughout your body, especially near your small blood vessels and near epithelial tissue—coverings such as linings of the airways or skin. Connective tissue binds together and supports other tissues and organs. It includes various kinds of fibrous tissue, fat, bone, and cartilage.

The IgE antibodies remain attached to the mast cells. Now the mast cells resemble little hand grenades, packed with ammunition (histamine and other allergy mediators). All it will take is a new invasion of the allergen to pull the trigger. In our example the cat allergen would finally activate these grenades and set off all those miserable symptoms of allergy— sneezing, runny nose, teary eyes. This stage of the allergy process is characterized by acute symptoms.

The IgE antibodies are especially designed to recognize and attach to the specific allergen that led to their creation. Like all antibodies, IgE molecules are shaped like the letter Y. Their base attaches to the mast or basophil cells and their arms extend outward. When invading allergens attach to at least two IgE antibodies, the grenade is triggered, and a cascade of chemicals is released in your body.

The most important of these, of course, is histamine, which dilates blood vessels, causes redness and, in extreme cases, shock. Histamine can also constrict the bronchial tubes to impair breathing, and this is why some allergic people develop asthma.

Histamine also irritates nerve endings, causing itching and pain, and stimulates the production of mucus in the respiratory system.

Then, there are the eosinophils, blood cells once thought to simply accumulate at the site of inflammation that occurs later on in the allergic reaction. Now we know they are active participants and they are sometimes called "allergy cells." In response to activation by mast cell mediators, eosinophils expand the inflammatory response. This results in more inflammation. If exposure to the allergen is constant, chronic inflammation can result.

SENSITIZATION AND EXPOSURE TO ALLERGENS

Exposure to allergens over a significant period of time is a major factor in developing an allergy. For example, getting a dose of cat allergen every day might take weeks or months. Seasonal pollen might take two to three seasons. During this time, you have no symptoms. You play with the cat and feel fine, but unfortunately, cells in your immune system are busy producing lots of IgE antibodies against the cat allergen. When the level becomes sufficiently high, symptoms develop.

The One-Two Punch of an Allergic Response

Your allergy response is usually composed of several phases.

Sensitization, as mentioned, is the initial exposure to an allergen and it leads to the production of
allergen-specific IgE antibodies in your immune
system. Sometimes people react only after multiple
exposures, often over years. People often develop
allergies to their pets years after they've brought
them home. A child with a cat at home may be
okay, but then he goes off to college, where there is
no cat, and his immune system adapts. When that
child comes home he is suddenly allergic to the cat.
If the immune system sees the allergen every day it
can sometimes tolerate it, but, after the allergen's
long absence, the immune system will overreact
when it sees it again. In another example, one can
have a severe allergic reaction to penicillin even
after taking it many times without adverse reaction.
One woman developed an allergy to penicillin after
previously receiving it 19 times with no reaction.

In most cases it is not clear why the immune system picks a specific time to overreact. People always
say, "Why now?" In some cases allergies follow an
infection of the airways, such as a bad cold or bron-
chitis. This may disrupt the lining, allowing more
allergens to get beyond the outer layer "epithelial"
airway barrier. Thus, a larger amount can get to the
immune system just below the epithelial barrier.

The early-phase reaction occurs within minutes of
exposure of the IgE antibody to the allergen and

causes the release of mediators such as histamine. Symptoms such as sneezing, runny nose, congestion, and itchy eyes peak rapidly, then gradually clear over a period of up to two hours because the mediators causing the early response have worn themselves out. In this calm phase, those mediators that will cause the late response are in the process of being formed.

The late-phase reaction can occur hours after exposure and reflects the influx of inflammatory cells (eosinophils). In this phase symptoms take longer to peak and persist longer. As a result of initial exposure to the allergen your nose becomes "primed"—it is more responsive to less stimulation. For example, if it takes 1,000 grains of pollen to bother you on the first day of pollen season, several weeks later it takes only 100 grains. Your allergy symptoms may also be aggravated by nonallergic factors, such as pollutants, irritant odors, cigarette smoke, and weather conditions. We'll say more about this later.

The Age When Allergies Begin

Allergies usually show up early in life, mostly before we are 20, with a large number of people developing them while they are children. Teenagers, more than any other age group, are prone to develop rhinitis. About 30 percent of adolescents suffer from both allergic and nonallergic rhinitis, compared with 10 percent of the total population. Twice as many young boys as girls get allergies, but by middle age the gender differences equalize. This may relate to hormonal effects on the development of the respiratory system. You can develop allergies at any age, though symptoms may diminish as you get older. Allergies wax and wane substantially and may disappear. However, exposure to new allergens, such as on a job where latex is airborne, may induce allergies later in life.

Allergic Rhinitis (a.k.a. Hay Fever)

Allergic rhinitis can also be triggered by seasonal pollen allergies as well as indoor allergens like animal proteins, mold, and the droppings of cockroaches or house dust mites. These are perennial or year-round allergies. Many people have both seasonal and perennial allergies; thus, they have chronic allergic rhinitis. Most people are allergic to more than one allergen, but if they are allergic to only one, it is usually dust mites.

Allergic rhinitis is an inflammation of the mucous membranes of your nose, which is commonly called hay fever. This is a misnomer, by the way, because hay is really a grass and there is no fever associated with allergies. Because hay is harvested in the fall, the symptoms were associated with hay. Fall allergy symptoms are actually due to weed pollens. It has also been called "rose fever" because spring symptoms due to tree pollen came at the same time that the roses were blooming.

In the Midwest and eastern United States about 75 percent of seasonal rhinitis is from ragweed, 50 percent from grass, and about 10 percent from tree pollen. This adds up to more than 100 percent because sensitivities overlap. About 5 to 10 percent of allergic people are allergic to all three kinds of pollen. About 25 percent are allergic to both ragweed and grass pollens.

Seasonal or perennial symptoms from airborne allergens can include:

- sneezing
- congestion
- runny nose
- itchiness in your nose, eyes, roof of your mouth, throat, and even deep inside your ears
- postnasal drip
- mouth breathing
- hoarseness
- snoring
- fatigue
- watery and red eyes
- nosebleed
- dry nose
- loss of sense of smell

HOW YOUR NOSE WORKS

What you see on your face is not all you get. Most of your nose is inside your head, between your eyes, above your mouth, and below your brain. This inner nasal cavity is a fairly complex area, but the parts you hear about most are the sinuses, the septum, and nasal membranes. Under this nasal membrane there's a rich supply of nerve cells, blood vessels, glands, and your lymph system, yellowish fluid that circulates through your body like blood, and helps protect you from infection.

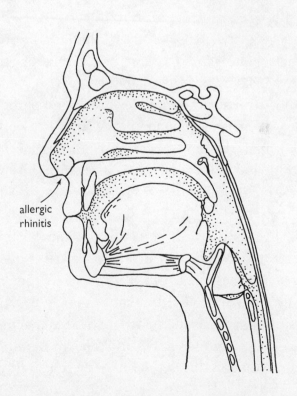

allergic
rhinitis

When the interior of your nose is too dry or you are ill, cracks can develop in this protective lining. Allergens get in through the normal lining of your nose, but if there are "cracks" they can get in more easily.

Multiple ridges (turbinates) in your nose do provide increased surface area to warm, humidify, and filter air before it gets to your lungs. Your nose prepares the air you breathe so it can enter your lungs. It warms up the cold air to body temperature very quickly. It also humidifies the air you breathe. This is one reason breathing through your nose is healthier than breathing through your mouth.

To have a normal sense of smell, regular air flow is needed across the olfactory (smell) cells in your nose. This only works if your nose is not clogged.

Your nose traps and eliminates unwanted particles and gases. Particles larger than a grain of salt rarely make it through the nose. Some gases like ozone, sulfur dioxide, and formaldehyde are absorbed by the gel layer of the lining and then swept clear by the mucus that leaves your nose. This clearing-out process is like sweeping your nose clean. Particles trapped in the back of your nose are swallowed. Others are swept toward your nostrils where they dry up and get blown out with a sneeze or by blowing your nose. Foreign agents, such as viruses or bacteria, are trapped by enzymes and antibodies in the lining of your nose that are designed to kill these bad guys.

Your nose also has a particular operating cycle. Every one to four hours the membranes on one side of your nostrils swell with blood while those on the opposite side empty out. You don't usually notice this cycle until something twitches your nose, such as a cold, allergy, or addiction to nasal sprays that exaggerates or prolongs the cycle.

WHY YOU SNEEZE

A sneeze occurs when the inside of your nose swells up, sort of like a blown-up balloon. When an allergen or an irritant like a piece of dust gets blown inside and hits the swollen lining, you sneeze. You may sneeze when the wind blows or a door opens or even if a strong odor wafts in your direction.

Do you sneeze if you are asleep? And how would you know? Usually, you get a reprieve at night when you are asleep. In most bedrooms, there is no airflow at night, thus we rarely sneeze during the night unless you are sleeping by an open window in pollen season. You are not walking around stirring up dust, so no particles get up your nose. The lining of your nose tends to be even more swollen when you are lying down, but the lack of a breeze protects you from sneezing. Even with air-conditioning, there is generally a filter, so particles get stirred up only if the unit is turned off for a while in a dusty room. In that case, the first blast of air may throw particles at your nose. When you first get up and throw off the covers, or open the closets, you may have a sneezing fit. You've just disturbed the sedentary dust particles.

Do You Have an Allergy or Just a Hyperactive Nose?

Lots of people come to an allergist convinced they have allergies. They complain of sneezing or runny nose when they enter a certain type of environment, or go to a certain region. This is very common. Quite often, they don't have allergies at all although they have rhinitis symptoms that are very similar to allergies.

Before you begin to treat your "allergies," you should first be sure you have allergies. This is clearly the first step in evaluation. You may think you have allergies, but the symptoms may have a different cause. For example, if you sneeze or wheeze when you use perfume, or hang around a smoke-filled room, this does not mean you are allergic to these substances. The nervous system in your nose may be confused. About half the people who think they are allergic really have a hyperactive nose. Irritants differ from allergens in that they don't produce a reaction in your immune system.

If your nose runs in winter when you are outside, this is from a nervous nose. Your nasal glands are responding to the cold by producing water. Then there is gastro-nasal reflex, when a distended stomach—eating too much—makes your nose run. So you do not know if you have an allergy without further investigation or testing.

To further confuse you, it is possible to have both allergic and nonallergic rhinitis. In fact, allergies can contribute to the nonallergic condition. Consider a spectrum: one end is nonallergic and the other end is allergic. Between these two poles, there are degrees of overreaction—and there's lots of overlap.

NONALLERGIC RHINITIS

Rhinitis is an inflammation of the mucous membranes of your nose, but it is not always caused by allergy. That's why it's a good idea to understand what else can cause it and how your nose responds to allergens as well as irritants.

Nonallergic rhinitis usually afflicts adults more than children and causes year-round symptoms, especially nasal congestion, stuffiness, or headaches. If you also have a very runny nose, the condition is often referred to as *vasomotor rhinitis*. Although medications cannot completely relieve symptoms, your doctor may prescribe decongestants or a steroid nasal spray to lessen symptoms. Interestingly, regular exercise can also be helpful. Doctors don't know why this is, but perhaps good physical conditioning helps the condition of the nose, too.

Irritants. Examples of airborne irritants are tobacco smoke, aerosols, paint, perfumes, cleaning products, room deodorizers, insecticides, or other strong odors or fumes. These are not allergens but can cause similar symptoms.

Weather changes. All types of rhinitis—including allergic—are aggravated by changes in the weather, especially if they are abrupt and dramatic. People with this type of sensitive nose can adapt to hot and humid or cold and dry but *not* to rapidly changing weather. This condition is partially responsive to nasal sprays. (See medications in chapter 8.)

Changes in the environment such as air pressure variations or weather shifts can also cause a type of non-allergic rhinitis, called eosinophilic nonallergic rhinitis. It is named after the blood cell—the eosinophil—that distinguishes it from other forms of nonallergic rhinitis. This type of rhinitis behaves like allergic rhinitis in that it causes frequent, recurrent bouts of sneezing and a runny nose. It is generally responsive to steroid nasal sprays.

Drug reactions. When over-the-counter deconges-tants and nasal sprays are used in excess—usually more than twice a day for three consecutive days—rhinitis medicamentosum occurs. This is called rebound congestion, or nasal spray addiction. These sprays shrink the lining of the nose so you feel clearer and more open momentarily, but when the spray wears off, your nose becomes more swollen than it was to begin with. This form of rhinitis causes severe nasal congestion. Treatment is to stop using the offending nasal spray, but usually temporary use of a steroid nose spray is also necessary.

Hormones. Any change of hormones in women, especially during puberty, menstruation, and pregnancy, can be associated with rhinitis. Hypothyroidism can also be a cause. When the symptoms are traced to a deficiency of thyroid hormone, medication can help.

Infections. A viral or bacterial infection of the nose or sinus is termed infectious or neutrophilic rhinosinusitis. This form of rhinitis is often associated with sinus pain, headache, and yellow-green mucus discharge. Treatment includes decongestants and nasal saline solution. If it is caused by a bacterial infection, antibiotics are necessary.

Structural abnormalities. If you were born with a small or crooked nasal passage or if you have broken your nose, you may have a nasal septum that is deviated to one side producing structural rhinitis. This can produce year-round congestion that usually affects one side of the nose more than the other. Surgery can help to correct this abnormality. (Sometimes, people with allergies also have structural abnormalities that exacerbate their allergies.)

Nasal polyps. Symptoms of rhinitis can also be caused by nasal polyps—benign growths in the mucous membrane of the nose—that can cause congestion and loss of sense of smell. They provoke symptoms year-round and frequently first develop between the ages of 20 and 40. Nasal polyps may be associated with aspirin sensitivity and asthma, and may cause recurrent sinusitis. Decongestants or corticosteroid nasal sprays or pills may give temporary relief. Nasal polyps can be surgically removed, but they have a tendency to return.

Allergic Conjunctivitis

Many allergic people have eye symptoms that can occur alone but are usually associated with nasal symptoms. Your eyes get red, tear, and itch intensely. These eye symptoms are part of the overall effect, but are technically called allergic conjunctivitis.

Those hyperactive mast cells are not only in your nose, but also in the clear mucous membrane lining the inner surface of your eyelid, and covering the front part of your eyeball, called the conjunctiva. When allergens get into your eye, histamine and other chemicals are released by these mast cells. This causes the blood vessels in the conjunctival lining to swell so your eye gets red, fluid leaks out, and the conjunctiva lining swells more. This can look like a coating of clear bumpy Jell-O over your eye, sparing the colored circle in the center, the iris. Thus, your eyes tear and often itch or swell.

The same allergens that spark your rhinitis in the spring, summer, or fall—airborne allergens such as grass, tree, and weed pollens and molds—can induce conjunctivitis. The main culprit is tree pollen. Perennial allergic conjunctivitis persists throughout the year and is usually triggered by indoor allergens such as dust mites, animal dander, and indoor molds.

About 22 million people in the United States suffer from allergic conjunctivitis. It is one of the most common forms of ocular allergy and often occurs in the fall. Allergic conjunctivitis can be disabling, and you need to take precautions to avoid allergens when possible and treat the condition with medication.

Some conjunctivitis is caused by infection and this, too, is common. There are two other types of allergic conjunctivitis.

Atopic Keratoconjunctivitis. This is associated with eczema or a rash on the eyelid and face. This type can occur in adolescence or early adulthood, particularly if there is a history of allergic rhinitis. In this condition the symptoms include

- red, oozing lesions of skin around the eye
- mucus discharge
- burning
- tearing
- corneal ulcer
- cataract
- photophobia (an aversion to light)

Vernal conjunctivitis is an ocular allergy that shows up with chronic inflammation in both eyes and commonly occurs in spring and fall. It is more common in boys and if left untreated, the scarring can lead to vision loss. This, too, frequently occurs in people with a history of allergic rhinitis or asthma. Symptoms include

- intense itching
- photophobia
- blurred vision
- stringy, ropy mucus discharge

If you experience these symptoms, you need to have your doctor refer you to an allergist and ophthalmologist, so both physicians can help to manage the condition.

The First Step to Relief:
Keep a Symptom Diary

The first step in any allergy treatment is to identify the allergen. It may be perfectly obvious. You go near a cat and sneeze, or a sudden pollen blitz may leave your eyes and nose running like Niagara Falls. But often, it's not so obvious. For example, if whenever you go to bed, your nose gets stuffed and you begin to sneeze, you need to figure out if you are allergic to dust mites in your bedding or if pollen is coming in your window. Think about the circumstances. If you live in a warm, damp climate or your house is near water or it has a damp basement, there could be dust mites there. However, if you live in a dry place, if there is a chronic leak in the wall of your bedroom, or carpeting covering a concrete floor (which traps moisture), then dust mites could be on hand. A damp basement may bring on symptoms, but you need to find out if you are allergic to mold or dust mites— both allergens often inhabit damp places.

Keep a diary to record time and circumstances. The most efficient way is to record your symptoms. It's better than relying on memory. After a month, you may have some clues and see a pattern.

- What are your symptoms?
- When do they occur, seasonally or all year?
- If they are seasonal, when do they occur?

- If you have symptoms all year, is there any difference at a certain time of year, winter or summer, or change of seasons?
- Is there any association between your symptoms and different locations, such as the city or the country? What about at the beach or in the mountains?
- Is there any association between your symptoms and various exposures such as animals, moldy places, or irritant odors?
- How long do the symptoms last?
- Is there anything you can do to relieve them?

Once some patterns emerge, or you identify any factor that increases your symptoms, such as exposure to dust, you can begin to take steps to limit your vulnerability. First, you can try to avoid the situation and allergen. Or you can also take an allergy medication before you are exposed to the allergen. The following chapters will help you do this.

Some Risk Factors You Can Change

Can you do anything to avoid allergies? Well, you cannot do much about your genetic programming. But you can avoid some risks. You can live at a high altitude where it is too dry for dust mites if you have that allergy. You can choose to live in a rural area and avoid air pollution if that is a factor.

Where you have most control, of course, is your level of awareness, level of exposure, and what you do to treat your symptoms.

ALLERGY CHECKLIST

✓ You inherit the genetic programming that makes you allergic from one or both parents.

✓ You do not become allergic until you are exposed to particular allergens over a period of time.

✓ Allergies usually begin in the early years of life but can begin at any time.

✓ Allergies wax and wane over your lifetime.

✓ Symptoms can begin right after exposure or hours later.

✓ Allergic rhinitis is commonly known as hay fever (a misnomer).

✓ Allergic rhinitis and allergic conjunctivitis symptoms usually occur together but can occur separately.

✓ Nasal symptoms may not be from allergies.

✓ Keeping a diary of your symptoms can help to identify your allergies.

2

POLLEN AND THE MATING SEASONS OF PLANTS

Think about it! If the wind didn't carry pollen from tree to tree and weed to weed, we would soon have a barren landscape. That's the positive point of view. The allergy-prone might prefer the negative spin: if the wind didn't carry all that pollen around we would have nothing to sneeze at. Bob Dylan wrote a wonderful song called "Idiot Wind," which is very deep and has nothing to do with allergies, but it's the kind of line you think of with a raised fist to the pollen-filled skies.

Most garden flowers don't trigger allergies because their pollen is too big to be airborne and too big to get into your lower airways. That's why bees are required to spread the pollen to other plants. But the small, light, dry pollens of many trees, grasses, and low-growing weeds are easily disseminated by the wind. These microscopic, powdery granules are less than the width of an average human hair and when they form clouds, they wreak havoc on the allergic people in the area.

Pollens are tiny, egg-shaped male cells of flowering plants necessary for fertilization. This frenzied plant-mating covers the entire globe at one time or another, and in some places it can go on forever. They are only present when the plant "flowers." No one's allergic to any other part of the plant, whether it's a tree, grass, or weed, with the exception of certain plants like poison ivy where contact with the leaves can cause skin allergy. "Flowers" on grass and weeds and many trees are not something you pick for their beauty and put in a vase on your table. These flowers are the sprouting fuzzy tops you see when the grass or weeds grow to a certain height. For example, a weed-strewn lot that is untended will have plenty of these feathery-looking tops. These are the flowers that produce the pollen that's blowing in the wind.

The pollen season generally begins in early spring and lasts through the fall. But this varies with regions and sometimes, even with plants. Trees pollinate earliest, from late February through May, although this may fluctuate in different locations. Grasses follow next in the cycle, beginning pollination in May and continuing into mid-July, but lasting all year in the South. Weeds usually pollinate in the late summer and early fall. These pollination periods do not vary greatly from year to year, but weather conditions can affect the amount of pollen in the air at any given time. (More on this later.)

Pollen is a long-distance allergen and frequent flyer. It can travel 300 miles on the prevailing winds. In the United States those winds blow from the West Coast to the East Coast, so living on the West Coast may save you from some sneezing because you have clear air from the Pacific and because the pollen is blowing away from you. However, pollen is not spread evenly through the air, but travels in clumps. You can walk down the street and all of a sudden have a sneezing fit because a breeze has just blown a batch of pollen from the trees overhead—even from one big tree ripe with pollen. But on the next block it may not be so bad. (Scientists have known about this wind and traffic pattern for years, but while tracking the patchy nuclear fallout from Chernobyl, they were able to measure it more accurately.)

Tree Pollen: It Doesn't Take a Forest

In the winter you should be able to walk through the woods or over a golf course without a sneeze or wheeze. But when the trees are in mating season, then even one robust tree could send you reeling when it spews its pollen.

While tree pollen accounts for only about 10 percent of allergies, it can be fierce when it occurs. It also tends to produce allergic conjunctivitis—itchy, watery eyes—more than other pollens. Tree pollen is the first seasonal allergen to appear, usually in early spring. (Trees may be dangerous to your allergies in the fall, too, when leaves on the ground become moldy.) Most tree pollen can induce allergies but certain trees are more potent than others, such as birch and oak in the Northeast and mountain cedar in the Southwest. Here are some of the trees causing allergies most of the time.

BIRCH TREES

Birch trees are the prime pollen problems in the northern United States and also in northern Europe (see chapter 13 on travel). In fact, most people allergic to tree pollen are allergic to birch. It is the number one culprit tree pollen in Alaska. In Austria, as many as 80 percent of people allergic to pollen are sensitive to pollen of the birch tree. The reason birch pollen is so powerful is that it contains some irritating proteins. Fortunately, the birch pollen season is short, lasting about two weeks.

The trees begin releasing pollen about two days before leaves emerge from buds. The concentration of pollen is greatest about three days after the leaves come out. The birch tree produces "catkins," clusters of tiny flowers that look like caterpillars. These can release millions of pollen grains. Most pollen falls within 20 feet of the tree, although much of it becomes airborne.

Silver birch, another species, is native to North America, and like the alder, likes to grow on river-banks.

THE MIGHTY OAK

Oak trees can account for more than a third of all the pollen in some regions. They pollinate from February through June (depending on the species), because oaks grow all over the country in a variety of climates. In the South, live oaks and white oaks polli-nate earlier, from February through April. Red oaks pollinate a bit later, from March through May. In the Northern states, oak pollen blows around in May and June.

Oak trees grow in all states except Alaska and Hawaii. There is a greater diversity of oak trees in the Southern states. Texas alone has more than 40 species. Oak pollen cross-reacts with birch tree pollen, so if both are around, your symptoms can be compounded.

ELM TREES

Elm trees, found mostly in the eastern half of the United States, are also prolific pollen producers, although Dutch elm disease has killed off great num-bers of these trees. If the winter is mild, pollen matures earlier in the spring. Pollination is intense but quick. Some trees release their pollen load over a two- to three-day period. Pollen appears from late

January into early March, depending on locale and climate. Some species of elm, however, pollinate in the late summer or early fall.

CEDAR TREES

The mountain cedar tree is the predominant tree in west and south Texas and the main culprit of allergies in Cedar Valley, named for the abundance of these trees, and the Texas hill country. Residents report seeing great clouds of pollen rising from the trees. These clouds look like smoke from fires. If you live in Texas, you may face a winter pollen attack from the cedar tree, which is abundant in that state. Though most trees pollinate in spring, cedars pollinate in December, January, and February and are the only plant allergen airborne at that time. A member of the cypress family, it is widely grown in Texas, especially in Austin and San Antonio.

The numbers of these trees have increased dramatically over the past 200 years because of the impact of controlling natural wildfires, which would normally limit the number and size of the trees. It is a prolific pollen producer and during peak seasons, pollen counts are high even miles from the trees.

Texans are not the only sufferers. Colorado and New Mexico are also rich in cedar. In fact, because of the large allergy problem in Albuquerque, the city banned the growing, selling, or planting of cedar trees, slapping fines of up to $500 on violators.

Farther north, related trees, such as the Rocky Mountain cedar, pollinate later, usually starting late in February or early March, but go on pollinating into June. However, the pollen counts are not so dramatic there.

White and red cedar trees in the Northeast and South also spew pollen, but not in such large quantities.

EVERGREENS IN NEW ENGLAND

For many years, while people complained that pine trees and other conifers (evergreens) were causing their seasonal rhinitis, it was often attributed to other causes. The pollen of pine is considered too large to get into the airways and it is covered with a waxy substance that covers up the allergens. Studies in the late 1980s and 1990s, however, showed through skin tests that some people are allergic to this type of tree pollen. Perhaps the waxy coating does not entirely block out the allergens. This type of tree pollen is a problem in New England, where most of the land is covered with conifers that pollinate from April through June. In fact, the allergen load is much higher than ragweed concentration in the autumn months. The Pollen and Mold Study Group of the New England Society of Allergy has been studying this allergen and reports that much of the pollen load in late May and June is from eastern white pine, the predominant conifer in that region.

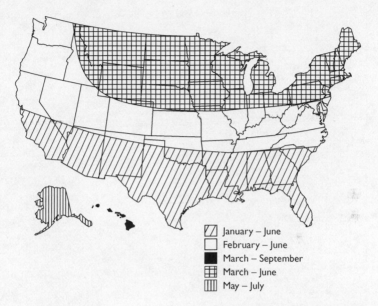

⧄	January – June
☐	February – June
■	March – September
⊞	March – June
⦀	May – July

Seasonal Tree Pollen Distribution

LESS ABUNDANT POLLINATORS

The box elder tree found in the Midwest is a potent allergen unlike the rest of the maple family, and many other trees produce pollen that may cause people to have allergic symptoms. In general, they are less abundant or less potent than those already mentioned. In Florida, palm trees produce pollen all year long, but palm pollen is not considered as allergenic as that of some other trees—unless, of course, you happen to be more sensitive. Cypress trees found in the South have a short pollen season from January to March or April.

Here are all the trees to which you could be allergic:

- Ash
- Alder
- Beech
- Birch
- Box Elder (maple)
- Elm
- Cottonwood
- Fir
- Hazelnut
- Hickory
- Juniper
- Maple
- Mesquite
- Mountain cedar
- Mulberry
- Oak
- Olive
- Pecan
- Pine
- Poplar
- Spruce
- Sweet gum
- Sycamore
- Walnut
- Willow

Grass Pollen: Fields of Allergens

Grass pollen accounts for about 50 percent of allergy symptoms. It is the biggest contributor to late spring and early summer airborne pollen allergies. The green stuff also accounts for about a quarter of the vegetation on the planet. It is found in mountains and deserts, around the water, between cracks in the sidewalks, everywhere.

Pollen is from the fuzzy top that sprouts when grass grows tall. It becomes airborne from wind blowing through it as well as raking, mowing, and simply walking on it. Even if you cut the grass before it flowers, there may be grass pollen elsewhere in the region that will affect you.

BLUEGRASS

Kentucky bluegrass conjures up images of thoroughbred horses grazing in sunny pastures, and indeed, 90 percent of this grass is found in wild pastures. It's estimated that bluegrass accounts for most of the pollen in the eastern United States during the first half of the season compared with all other grasses combined. In Europe, too, bluegrass produces the most pollen. And a very aggressive invader it is. It will crowd out other grasses and produces abundant seed. This makes it very useful commercially for landscapers and builders. Bluegrass is a good sod builder and used for lawns everywhere because its turf is dense, and has deep roots.

TIMOTHY GRASS

The other potent grass is timothy, a tall grass and the nation's most commercially important perennial grass. It is cultivated for hay in at least four times the amount of all other hay grasses combined. Timothy is widely grown in the Northeast, west to the Missouri River, and south to Missouri and Virginia. It is also grown in irrigated areas of the West. It grows best in meadows and grassy parks and canyon bottoms.

Timothy is two to four feet tall and sheds large

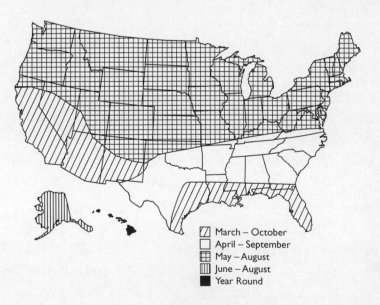

Seasonal Grass Pollen Distribution

amounts of pollen, primarily in the morning hours. Depending on the region, peak pollen season is between May and October. When this grass is dried out for use as hay, lots of pollen is still trapped in it, and this is why hay can be a problem in the fall.

BERMUDA GRASS

Bermuda is a coarse grass found in the South. Most of the lawns in Florida are planted with this grass, but beware, because the golf courses are usually bluegrass.

Northern grasses generally cross-react with one another. Coarse grass in southern regions, such as Bermuda, doesn't cross-react with Northern grasses, so you may not have symptoms there. Perhaps you want to spend the early summer pollen season in Florida, rather than the North.

You may opt for concrete landscaping to avoid grass pollen, but if your neighbors have lawns, your efforts will be in vain. In late spring and early summer, pollinating grasses pull the allergic rhinitis symptom trigger. There are more than 1,200 types of grasses, but only a few cause allergic reactions. The main ones are the three mentioned, but others include orchard, sweet vernal, and red top.

Ragweed: The King of Pollens

Ragweed is said to be the number one cause of allergic rhinitis, responsible for 75 percent of that condition in the United States. In the Midwest, ragweed is called "king." Not only is ragweed pollen extremely potent, it comes from one of the ugliest and most putrid-smelling plants on earth. This hairy, coarse-looking plant with unattractive flowers is related to the sunflower plant. It is known as ambrosia, its scientific name meaning food for the gods. Its popular name, from the ragged appearance of its leaves, seems much more appropriate.

Ragweed grows in newly disturbed soil, in ditches, in dry fields, pastures, construction sites, and even in your garden or yard. It grows in great profusion along the roads and highways.

This ugly weed also gets turned on by a hostile growing environment. In fact, the more hostile the environment, the more pollen the plant will produce. Stress, lack of rain, diesel fumes, all serve to stimulate the weed into procreation. This way it skimps on foliage and directs its resources into the bloom that produces pollen. Ragweed is so tough that it resists all attempts to wipe it out.

The short ragweed plant can bloom and spew pollen into the air when only a few inches tall. The giant version of the plant can be 12 feet tall. A ragweed plant lives only one season, but it produces up to one billion pollen grains. Even if the pollen count is as low as 20 grains per cubic meter of air, it can trigger an allergic reaction.

But remember pollen is passive. It only goes where the wind blows it, so a calm day should not bother you. Once the wind carries it off, it flies in whenever you open a door or window. It comes in on your clothing and shoes and on your pets. Ragweed pollen is so small, it can get into your house through the tiniest cracks. Pollen samples have been found 400 miles out to sea and two miles high in the air. Because ragweed pollen is carried such long distances, efforts to stamp it out from any one region remain futile. It drifts in from miles away.

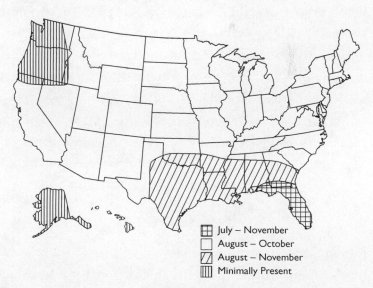

July – November
August – October
August – November
Minimally Present

Seasonal Ragweed Pollen Distribution

Ragweed grows during hot, dry weather. If the hot, dry weather is prolonged, then the plant keeps producing and the amount of pollen dispersed by the plant tends to be very high. Peak pollen time for ragweed is mid-August through November, or whenever the first frost occurs. The season usually peaks in mid-September in many areas of the country.

A native of North America, ragweed was unknown in Europe until very recently. It's now been reported in central France, Hungary, Austria, Northern Italy, and Switzerland. People who come here to work in the United States from Europe often develop this allergy after two or three years. They have to go through at least one season to get exposure. One woman seemed to become sensitized in her first ragweed season in the United States, but it turned out she had made a visit to the U.S. in September the previous year and had become sensitized then.

Ragweed is most common in the Northeast and Midwest. Tulsa has the dubious distinction as the worst city for ragweed in the United States, according to the latest studies. In this country, only the Northwest is spared.

Other Bad Weeds

Ragweed is the pollen most responsible for late summer and autumn rhinitis in North America, but other weed pollens can trigger allergic rhinitis symptoms.

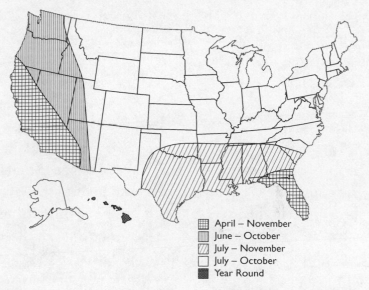

April – November
June – October
July – November
July – October
Year Round

Seasonal Weed Pollen Distribution

SAGEBRUSH

Giant sagebrush is a significant cause of allergic rhinitis throughout the Western United States. It is a woody perennial weed suited to the arid areas of the Rocky Mountains and Great Basin. It is the most abundant Western shrub and the dominant vegetation for great expanses in the mountain states. It produces so much pollen that when the wind blows, you can see small yellow clouds overhead. The season is between July and September in the north central and northwest areas of the country, and in August to October in the Southwest.

It grows in areas with elevations of up to 8,000

feet. It's normally about three feet high but can grow as high as ten feet. The bark is grayish brown and stringy and the leaves are silvery blue-gray. Giant sagebrush is often eaten by livestock because it has a high protein content.

TUMBLEWEED

Tumbleweed gets around. The loose plants bounce around the desert Southwest like beach balls. They are such a symbol of the West, memorialized in song and movies, that most of us think of them as native to the region. We are wrong, however. These plants are actually interlopers and it is suspected they came to this country in the 1870s with Ukrainian farmers. The real name of these weeds is Russian thistle. Pollen grains of this weed have also been found on the Shroud of Turin in the Middle East, so they are newcomers to America. And they wreak havoc to allergy sufferers.

The weed is actually a relative of spinach, and desert animals love to snack on this plant. But it grows fast and forms a round mass of tough and prickly stems. It grows up to six feet high and twice that across. Low levels of pollination begin in the spring and gain momentum through the summer with peak levels in September. In late fall the mature plant breaks free and bounces along with the wind. It scatters its seeds everywhere. Its pollen shrouds the air of the Southwest.

Other weeds like kochia, which resembles tumble-weed, and pigweed add to the pollen infestation of the West.

DOCK WEED

Dock weed pollinates in late spring to early summer, unlike most weeds. The most intense pollination is from late April through May, but may persist well into the summer. In fact, in California and southern Florida, dock may pollinate all year long. Most dock weeds produce abundant pollen with counts as high as some grasses. The impact of this weed's pollen has been underestimated because its season overlaps with grass pollination.

There are many species of this weed found in the United States. Flowers of the *Rumex* type dock weed are pendulous, greenish, without petals, and wind pollinated. Flowers of curly dock are first yellow-green, then turn rosy and ultimately dark red-brown, stalks of which can be identified from a great distance in late summer.

How the Weather Affects Airborne Allergens

All types of rhinitis—including allergic—are bothered by changes in air pressure or weather shifts. Thunderstorms pull up grass pollen from the ground because of the negative air pressure, and this can increase rhinitis symptoms. When there are thunderstorms the number of asthmatics seen in emergency rooms increases.

One New York City woman's rhinitis symptoms always flared up before a summer thunderstorm. If the weather forecast called for thunderstorms, she learned to take preventive medications. Because doctors in many countries have noticed this thunderstorm phenomenon, some Australian medical researchers looked for some answers. They found that during pollen season, thunderstorms seem to sweep up the allergenic particles and concentrate them in a narrow band of air close to the ground. This is the storm's outflow. When this occurs, the concentration of airborne pollen increases from four to twelve times. According to researchers, as a thunderstorm passes over a field of grass, it draws the pollen grains up into the atmosphere and then forces them into a downdraft. This puts much more pollen at ground level—or very close to your nose.

We can't see grass pollen, but it travels hundreds of miles, so you can react if you are in a city or in a rural area covered with grass. The good news is that the heavy rain of a storm usually cleans the air and lowers pollen levels.

However, rain promotes growth, so after a period of rain, pollen is released in greater amounts. Birch tree pollen germinates with rain to produce pollen tubes. When leaves dry out, the tubes rupture and release large amounts of pollen.

Your allergy symptoms may often be minimal on days that are rainy, cloudy or windless, because pollen does not move about during these conditions. Hot, dry and windy weather signals greater pollen distribution and thus, increased allergy symptoms.

IS GLOBAL WARMING CHANGING THE POLLEN SEASON?

Many people suspect global warming may be extending the seasonal clock and thus, our allergy symptoms. So far there is not much proof. The amount and timing of pollen in the air depends on temperature and the amount of rain, which, at least in part, may be affected by global warming. However, fluctuations have occurred throughout history so we cannot isolate the effect of global warming.

In the spring of 2001, it was suddenly and unusually warm in New York City, coming on the heels of a prolonged and intense winter. This prompted the trees to pollinate seemingly overnight, driving up pollen levels to heights not seen in years. Cars were covered with yellow dust from falling pollen. At one counting station levels reached 6,790 grains of pollen per cubic meter of air. (Days later it fell to 35.) The National Allergy Bureau considers 15 to 89 particles to be moderate. Heat stimulates plants to pollinate, but sudden heat means every plant pollinates at once. Few allergy sufferers were ready for such a deluge. Normally, pollination comes on gradually, but we cannot blame global warming for this.

The Effect of Ozone and Pollution

On the other hand, increased ozone and pollution do have an effect on allergy symptoms. When the ozone level is up, your nose and lung airways become more sensitive and it takes less pollen to induce allergy symptoms. So, if global warming is increasing the ozone, then it does have some effect.

Ozone is the major harmful ingredient in smog. It is produced when gases or vapors from organic chemicals called hydrocarbons combine with nitrogen oxide compounds in the presence of sunlight. Hydrocarbon gases are released from a variety of sources such as refineries, gas stations, motor vehicles, chemical plants, and solvents.

When the ozone level is high, pollens are held in the air. Ozone can inflame and cause harmful changes in breathing passages, decrease the lung's working ability, and cause both coughing and chest pains. Ozone air pollution is found at unhealthful levels in nearly all of our major urban areas. It may affect millions of otherwise healthy Americans who, for reasons we don't yet understand, are especially sensitive to it.

The Lancet, a British medical journal, reported on studies from London and Cairo, showing that the acute inhalation of ozone significantly increases airway responsiveness and impairs lung function in both asthmatic and nonasthmatic people. By contrast, studies on nitrogen dioxide inhalation have shown inconsistent effects on lung function and airway responsiveness. Sulfur dioxide also leads to bronchoconstriction in both healthy and asthmatic people.

Exposure to a combination of sulfur dioxide and nitrogen dioxide in levels that are encountered in heavy traffic enhances the airway response to inhaled allergens. If you are exposed to this, and then also challenged by dust mites, you will have greater sensitivity to the mites.

Exercise makes you more vulnerable to the effects of ozone, too, because you take in more air, thus causing more symptoms and a reduced ability to breathe at relatively low ozone levels. Even at low levels, ozone has also been linked to an increase in hospital admissions and emergency room visits for respiratory problems.

Don't confuse the harmful ozone in the lower atmosphere with ozone in the upper atmosphere, which protects us from ultraviolet radiation.

DIESEL EXHAUST PARTICLES

Airborne pollens can bind to diesel exhaust particles (DEP) in the air and these exhaust particles affect the immune system response and the production of IgE. Studies by researchers from several groups including the University of Los Angeles School of Medicine, where smog and ozone is a critical problem, have found this to be true. In recent decades more diesel fuels are used by the trucking industry. In fact, 88 percent of all heavy-duty trucks now run on diesel fuel. Both human and animal studies have shown both short- and long-term effects of such exposure. The UCLA study, reported in 1997, showed that diesel extracts promoted a 16 times greater antigen-specific IgE response to ragweed than the allergen alone. So, by elevating IgE production, this allergen/diesel combination can increase your allergic airway symptoms.

MORE TRAFFIC AND MORE RAGWEED POLLEN

Motor vehicle pollution has been cited in the rapid increase of ragweed—the most potent allergen in the United States. The United States Department of Agriculture studied the effect of higher carbon dioxide levels that are associated with global warming on ragweed pollen. In the study released in 2000, researchers claimed the amount of pollen that an average ragweed plant produces might have doubled over the preceding four or five decades. We have more cars, more carbon dioxide (CO_2), and more ragweed. They predict another doubling by the end of the twenty-first century.

Investigators at the Johns Hopkins University School of Public Health, working with the USDA, are growing ragweed at three locations in Baltimore, chosen for their range in temperatures. Baltimore is typical of urban areas with heat islands and zones of high carbon dioxide concentrations, as well as part suburb, and part rural area. This ongoing experiment should show how global warming and higher CO_2 levels might already be increasing ragweed pollen counts, especially in cities, say these scientists.

Carbon dioxide stimulates the growth not only of ragweed, but 96 percent of all plant species capable of producing carbon, according to study author Lewis H. Ziska, Ph.D., a plant physiologist in the Climate Stress Laboratory of the USDA. Rising atmospheric carbon dioxide is an important factor in determining pollen levels.

Although less ragweed grows in cities, exposure to air pollutants such as ground-level ozone can make people more sensitive to ragweed pollen. As already mentioned, diesel exhaust particles stimulate IgE production in the upper respiratory mucous membrane. Thus, diesel fuel can also stimulate allergic reactions to pollen.

PARTICULATE MATTER

In recent years particulate matter (PM) has come to the attention of health researchers. These microscopic particles and tiny droplets of liquid are spewed into the air from the burning of fuels by industry and diesel vehicles and from earth-moving activities such as construction and mining. Larger particles can be stopped in your nose and upper lungs by your body's natural defenses. The smallest particles escape those defenses and go deep into the lungs, where they may become trapped. Exposure to PM can cause wheezing and other symptoms in people with asthma or sensitive airways. Particulate pollution has been linked to increased hospital admissions and ER visits for respiratory problems and to a substantial increase in premature deaths.

When sulfur-containing fuel is burned, primarily in power plants and diesel engines, it creates sulfur dioxide (SO_2). This can also change in the atmosphere into acidic particles and into sulfuric acid. It constricts air passages, making it a problem for people with asthma and for young children whose small lungs need to work harder than adult lungs. Even brief exposure—such as standing behind an idling bus—to relatively low levels of sulfur dioxide can cause an asthma attack.

Most chemicals find their way into the air but many are dispersed before they do any harm. Some are so common and widespread, however, that they build up in the air and become a health hazard. Toxic and cancer-causing chemicals can be inhaled directly or carried by small particles into the lungs. Millions of pounds of these chemicals are emitted into the air over our nation every year by motor vehicles and by both large and small industry.

So while pollution may not cause allergies, it does enhance their effect and in most cases it directly irritates the airways.

ALLERGY CHECKLIST

✓ Pollen from trees, grass, and weeds, is carried for hundreds of miles via the wind.

✓ Birch tree pollen is the prime tree allergen in the Midwest and Northeast.

✓ Mountain cedar pollen causes high incidence of allergies in Texas.

✓ Bluegrass and timothy grass are responsible for most allergies to grass pollen.

✓ Ragweed is the "king" of pollens in the Midwest.

✓ Sagebrush and tumbleweeds produce lots of allergens in the Southwest.

✓ A thunderstorm pulls up more pollen from the grass.

✓ High ozone levels make you more sensitive to allergens.

✓ Diesel emissions are adding to the amount of ragweed pollen.

3

STRATEGIES FOR MINIMIZING YOUR EXPOSURE TO AIRBORNE POLLEN

Most of us can't leave town during a particular pollen season. We have jobs and families. We have a life and it's not designed to coincide with the pollen count. And there's no place on earth anymore that's entirely free of allergens, unless you consider the polar region agreeable. Decades ago people with allergies moved to Arizona to escape the grass and weed pollens in the rest of the country. Guess what? The allergens came right along with them as they planted lawns and trees and gardens.

What do you do if you cannot leave the pollen or the pollution behind? Once you've identified the allergens, the next step is avoiding them at all costs. Well, at least as much as humanly possible.

Avoiding the allergens that make us miserable is the best single treatment, but the one that is least followed. The best scenario is to live in an air-conditioned house, go to work on air-conditioned transportation, and work in an air-conditioned environment. The air-conditioning units have filters that should remove most of the pollen. Remember they need to be cleaned regularly, and periodically new filters need to be inserted. If you can't remain in such protective environments, there are some ways you can cut down on exposure.

Know When to Go Out and When to Come In

How best to avoid airborne pollen depends on the time of day, the weather, and how far off the ground you are. This may be easier in an air-conditioned building than outdoors where you have less control, but there are some things you can do to protect yourself.

- Pollen levels are highest from early morning to midafternoon and again in the early evening. The hours between mid- and late afternoon are the best time to do your outdoor activities.
- Dew tends to weigh down pollen, but in the heat of the sun, the pollen dries and begins to rise. The air in midafternoon is relatively pollen free at ground level, but 20 stories up the pollen count may be higher.

- Highest pollen levels are in parks and meadows with lots of trees and grass.
- Ragweed pollen can travel far, but most falls close to the source. Don't jog on the side of the weedy road and close the windows of your car.

More Prevention Tips

At any time of day or night, you can do a great deal to minimize your exposure and your misery, such as keeping windows closed at night to prevent pollens or molds from drifting into your home. Also, keep car windows closed when traveling. Minimize outdoor activity on days when the pollen count is reported to be high or on windy days when more pollen is airborne. Take a shower after spending time outdoors to remove pollen that may be on your skin and hair. Of course, others you live with need to do the same.

WEAR A MASK

There was a time when seeing masked people jogging or mowing the lawn would make us think the aliens had landed. No longer. You need a very fancy respirator mask to block inhalation of allergens 1 to 5 microns in size, but a paper mask may screen out some, at least during allergy season or in periods when air pollution is particularly high. These inexpensive masks are available at any drug or hardware store. Keep a supply in your car, your office, and at home.

For better protection, you need a mask with a HEPA (high efficiency particulate arresting) filter in order to screen out minute allergens like pollen and mold. These are lighter in weight than respirator masks and you can reuse the filters and face piece. Lightweight latex straps secure the mask comfortably. It is designed not to interfere with your vision, so you can wear sunglasses to protect your eyes. (If you are allergic to latex, don't use this mask.) A complete kit with two filters sells for about $20. Two packs of replaceable filters cost about $7.

STAY IN YOUR SHADES

If you tend to get itchy, watery eyes from pollen attacks, wear big wraparound sunglasses to help block pollen from getting into your eyes. Contact lenses may present problems if pollen and irritants get under the lens; you may be better wearing regular eyeglasses during heavy pollen times. Sports stores or places where allergy products are sold have goggles that cover and protect your eyes. Again, be cautious if you are allergic to latex. (See chapter 8 for eye allergy remedies.)

WEAR NATURAL FIBERS

Pollen sticks to your clothing, hair, shoes, everything. Synthetic fabrics like polyester create an electrical charge when you move around and the fabric rubs against itself. The charge attracts pollen, which is also electrically charged. Natural fibers like cotton do not create this charge and also breathe better. They stay drier and less hospitable for moisture-loving mold, too. Dry your clothes in the dryer rather than on the clothesline during allergy season so you don't bring pollen into the house.

EXERCISE INDOORS OR BEFORE SUNRISE

When you exercise, you breathe in more air—and thus, more allergens. Do it at a time of day with less pollen. Breathe through your nose, not your mouth. Remember your nose is a filter. If it's plugged up it won't work. If it's so stuffy that you can't breathe properly, make sure you talk with your doctor about using medication first with nasal sprays or antihistamine that won't make you feel tired. (See chapter 8 for medications.)

In addition to avoiding pollen-showered parks or fields, steer clear of major highways and industries when you exercise. Chemicals from exhaust and from factory smokestacks can irritate nasal passages and make allergy symptoms worse. And remember all that ragweed along the highway! You don't need to become a couch potato and lock yourself up indoors with air-conditioning, but cut your risk. Hit the mall for your long power walk, rather than the side of the road with ragweed. Sign up for the gym during pollen season.

A woman in her twenties began running after a

period of relative inactivity. And as we all do when we suddenly decide to get back in shape, she overdid it. She began running in June near a field where grass was being cut. She inhaled huge quantities of grass pollen because exercise makes you breathe in more air. Previously, she had infrequent symptoms of allergic rhinitis. But because she was now exposing herself to the worst set of circumstances, she had a serious anaphylactic reaction of asthma and hives. When questioned later by her doctor, she admitted to being out of shape, running at the peak grass pollen season, and at the peak time of day in a place with a maximum amount of pollen. This combination of factors caused her to inhale larger amounts of grass pollen and resulted in the asthma and hives.

IN THE GARDEN

If you're allergic to plant pollens, it might be wise to choose a hobby other than gardening. However, if you like to garden, and even if you live in a home surrounded by attractive landscaping with plants, trees, and shrubs, it may be worthwhile learning something about the pollen habits of plants so you can cut down on vulnerability to symptoms.

According to Thomas Leo Ogren, author of *Allergy-Free Gardening*, you should stick to female plants and avoid introducing pollen-producing male plants into your garden. Although there is no scientific evidence that this will help your allergies, it might be worth thinking about. A landscaper could probably help you identify the most suitable plants.

If you are allergic to birch pollen, avoid having the trees near your house, since birch trees drop most of their pollen within 20 feet of the tree. Red maple and other trees are lower on the pollen potency scale and may be a wiser choice.

If you like to get up close and personal with plants in your garden, choose showy, flowering trees and shrubs such as apple and cherry trees and azaleas. They produce waxy pollen that's too heavy to ride the breeze. On the lawn, opt for nonpollinating ground cover such as myrtle and ivy rather than grass. (But if your neighbors within 100 miles have grass, then you will still be vulnerable.) During the spring grass season keep the grass short before it can sprout pollen-producing flowers.

Protect yourself as much as possible while working in your garden. Wear a mask when you dig around in the dirt, rake leaves, or mow the lawn. These activities stir up pollen (and mold). Check with your doctor about taking an antihistamine one hour ahead of time. (See chapter 8.)

Leave your outer work clothes outside and wash them before using again. Take a shower immediately and wash your hair. Allergens will land in your eyelashes and brows as well. Wash your hands and rinse out your eyes, if you tend to react to pollen.

What the Pollen Count Really Means

Pollen and mold levels are compiled by a variety of methods, and are reported as grains per cubic meter of air. These pollen counts can be affected by the type of device used to measure the pollen and where in the community the device is located. Many universities, medical centers, and clinics provide these counts on a voluntary basis.

The pollen counts that you hear on your radio and TV news are actually 24 to 36 hours old by the time they are broadcast. And pollen counts may vary widely from day to day during a season. So, the use of pollen counts in predicting severity of your allergy symptoms is somewhat limited. Remember pollen is not the only allergen you may be exposed to. While many people develop symptoms when pollen counts are 20 to 100 grains per cubic meter, your symptoms may also be affected by the intensity of your exposure to a particular allergen, your recent exposure to other allergens, and last but not least, your own level of sensitivity.

The National Allergy Bureau (NAB) is the nation's only pollen and mold counting network certified by the American Academy of Allergy, Asthma and Immunology (AAAAI). As a free service to the public, the NAB compiles pollen and mold counts from certified stations across the country and reports them to the media three times each week. But it's only available during pollen season. These counts are also available on the NAB page of the AAAAI Web site (AAAAI.org) and through the toll free number (800-0-POLLEN) from 8 A.M. to 8 P.M. every day.

Also on the Internet, you can find pollen.com (and other sites) for the most recent pollen count and other helpful information. If you plug in your own zip code, you'll find out if the pollen in your area is high (red), medium (green), or low (yellow). For instance, on one day in 2001 it listed New York City and Newark, New Jersey among the five worst cities in the country for allergy problems. The site is operated by Surveillance Data, Inc., a research company, that maintains a continuous running list of pollen counts in cities across the country.

Avoid Foods That Cross-react with Pollen

If you have allergic rhinitis, you may notice that when you eat certain foods your mouth becomes itchy or even swollen. This can extend to the back of your throat. People worry that they have food allergies, but certain foods contain allergens called profilins that cross-react with pollens. Your allergy system cannot tell the difference. This is a problem only with raw fruit and occasionally vegetables. Heating breaks down the culprit profilin, so you should eat only cooked, canned, or bottled versions of the fruit.

The most common oral allergy syndrome (OAS) reaction is sensitivity to apples and the peach and plum chemical family in people allergic to birch tree pollen. Sometimes they also react to melon. These symptoms are worse in spring when their allergy system is stimulated during pollen exposure. Sometimes they can tolerate eating the fruit in midwinter.

OAS is not the same as a serious food allergy and has not been associated with life-threatening reactions. However, if you have any reaction beyond the direct contact area, presume you may have a true food allergy. Such reactions range from hives to a life-threatening problem with breathing or a drop in blood pressure. If this happens, you must see an allergy specialist for evaluation. You will be advised to avoid the culprit food and carry an EpiPen.

Specific cross-reactions have been identified between tree, grass, and ragweed pollens and certain fruits and vegetables.

OAS symptoms will usually decrease or disappear with immunology treatment (allergy shots with extracts of the cross-reacting pollens). This stops the immune system from overreacting to the pollen. People with OAS also report that some improvement occurs with the use of regular doses of antihistamines.

Here are the common cross reactors:

Pollen allergy	Food to avoid
Birch tree	Apple, pear, peach, plum, cherry, nectarine, kiwi, celery, carrot, cantaloupe, honeydew, hazelnut

Pollen allergy	Food to avoid
Grass	tomato, kiwi
Ragweed	cantaloupe, honeydew, watermelon, chamomile tea, banana, sunflower

Some foods cross-react with latex allergen, and you'll find that information in chapter 10, which deals with allergies on the job. While it is impossible to avoid all seasonal airborne allergens, with some allergy savvy you can cut down the effects with as much avoidance as possible and by using your medications correctly. This information is in chapter 8.

ALLERGY CHECKLIST

✓ Pollen levels are highest in the morning and early afternoon and again in the evening.

✓ Pollen levels are lowest before the sun dries the dew and for a couple of hours between late afternoon and evening.

✓ The best way to avoid pollen is to stay in an air-conditioned environment.

✓ A HEPA mask can filter out allergens.

✓ Protect your eyes with wraparound sunglasses or goggles; don't wear contact lenses.

✓ Natural fibers attract less pollen than synthetics.

✓ Exercise indoors.

✓ Shower when you go inside after being out in a pollen environment.

✓ Daily pollen counts are 24 to 36 hours old before they are broadcast on the news.

✓ Avoid raw fruits and vegetables that cross-react with pollen.

4

MOLD SPORES: AIRBORNE MOST OF THE TIME

For many people with allergies, autumn is an especially bad time of the year. If you are allergic to both ragweed and mold, the fall is a one-two punch. On an average fall day in allergy season there may be more than 500 grains of ragweed per cubic meter of air, and ten times as many—5,000—spores of mold. While there is generally more mold in the air, ragweed is a more potent allergen. Unlike pollens, molds do not have a specific season, except perhaps in the Midwest grain-growing states. Molds thrive on these plants. Otherwise, they do tend to be most prolific in the fall when there is adequate dampness and a good source of food such as dead leaves.

Airborne mold levels are especially high in damp, shady spots with rotting wood or vegetation, on freshly cut lawns, fields, and pastures. You walk through this soil and trek it home where it sinks right into your carpets. Molds are present in almost every possible habitat, but tend to be highest in warm and humid weather, especially after a rain shower. They reach their peak in July in warmer states and October in the colder states. Mold spore levels in the air are particularly high just before a frost and again after the spring thaw. But molds can be found all year long outdoors in the South and on the West Coast.

Mold counts are not as reliable as pollen counts, as it is technically difficult to trap and count the spores. Also, mold spore levels are directly related to weather and vary more widely over the course of a day compared to pollen.

If your allergy symptoms are worse on rainy or damp days than on dry, sunny days, then you may well be allergic to mold spores.

THE VARIED LIFE OF MOLD SPORES

Molds are microscopic fungi related to mushrooms. There are thousands of varieties and they survive outdoors and indoors. They feed on other organic material, which they decompose in order to produce food for themselves. This is why, in temperate climates, your symptoms may not clear up after the first frost, because the frost kills all of the plants but spares the mold. As soon as there is a thaw, the mold will thrive on the dead foliage until the hard frost sets in. If there is no "hard frost" or cold winter where you live, you could have airborne mold all year round.

Disturbing a mold source, such as a compost heap or wallpaper on a damp wall, can disperse the spores into the air. These are tiny reproductive cells that become airborne and cause the allergy symptoms. Some release spores during the day, other at night. The spores differ in size, shape, and color among species, but each spore that germinates can give rise to new mold growth, which in turn can produce billions more spores.

Mold spores float in the air like pollen, and because they are present throughout the year in many states they are a perennial allergy problem as well as a seasonal one. Because spores are so small and they bypass all the normal safeguards in the nasal passages, they easily get into the lower respiratory tract and lungs.

There are many types of mold, but studies have shown that only a few are responsible for most of the airborne concentrations. These are alternaria, cladosporium, and aspergillus. Molds can only be identified if they are growing in a large mass. Otherwise they have to be viewed under a microscope in order to be identified. It has been difficult to study mold allergies because of the technical difficulties encountered in trying to grow them in a lab. As a result, mold extracts used for skin testing are less standardized.

People in some occupations have more exposure to mold and are at greater risk of developing allergies. In addition to grain farmers who grow wheat, oats, corn, or barley, others are vulnerable. Bakers, loggers, mill workers, and carpenters are at risk. So are wine makers and those who work in green-houses. On farms, grain bins and silos are likely places to find mold. For more about occupational allergens, see chapter 10.

How to Find Out If You Are Allergic to Mold

Most allergy symptoms are caused by outdoor mold even if you get symptoms while indoors. Outdoor molds can be found inside on floors, tracked in by shoes from outside. Mold in food or on bathroom tiles is usually not a source of allergy. If you have a water leak resulting in mold growth, however, this may cause symptoms.

People often think they are allergic to mold when they return to a summer home after the winter and develop nasal congestion or runny nose and sneez-ing. The house is musty and smells of mildew. In some cases, mold will be the culprit, in other cases dust mites may be the problem. (See chapter 5.) For the majority of people, their nose may simply be oversensitive to irritant odors.

First, ask yourself some of the following ques-tions. They may seem obvious, but if you begin to keep track, you may find out whether or not you are allergic to mold.

1. How do you feel on severely damp summer days?

2. Do your allergy symptoms flare up when you walk into a damp, musty house or basement? What about a barn or garage?

3. Do you feel uncomfortable on hayrides? Symptoms provoked by grass cutting or hay are often caused by mold, not pollen.

4. Do you notice symptoms when you walk through fallen leaves or when raking them? Fallen leaves become moldy very quickly.

5. Do you feel stuffy or sneeze when you work in a greenhouse or garden?

If you answer yes, try some simple tests yourself before you get tests from your doctor. Try breathing in the moldy area and the nonmoldy area. Do you feel a difference? Try to fix the problem first, such as a damp basement, and see if you get better.

There are ways to determine your response to mold by avoiding it and testing the mold itself.

TESTING FOR MOLD

If you see an allergy specialist, he or she may have you order special mold plates to test in your home. These are petri dishes full of agar jelly. You place them in suspect areas. If there is mold present, it will land on the plate and grow on the agar. The plates are then sent to a company for analysis. If there is a big growth of one mold, then your doctor can test you for an allergy to that mold.

Often outside molds are brought in on shoes and will stick to carpets, and this makes testing tricky to do. Sometimes we cannot tell if the mold is indigenous to the inside of the house or it came in from outside. Your doctor will advise you to put mold plates outside and in other areas for comparison as background controls.

Then you need to be tested yourself to see if your immune system reacts to that particular mold. Your doctor can do a blood test to confirm your suspicions. (See chapter 7 on getting allergy tests.)

The chief problem with mold allergen is that it is very difficult to grow in culture to provide material for research and for commercial production of allergy testing and treatment materials. For this reason mold allergen is not as well studied as, for example, pollen. We particularly lack data on indoor mold.

Getting Rid of Mold: Lower the Humidity

Allergy to indoor molds is a minimal problem compared to outdoor exposure. About 98 percent of allergy to airborne mold is caused by outside molds, and there is not much you can do about that, except to avoid activities in high risk areas, like walking through a pile of dead leaves.

If you are allergic to mold, the first step is to assess the extent of the mold and humidity around you. There are problems outside and inside your home to consider. There are some obvious clues to high humidity, such as sweating windowpanes in winter or paint peeling off a house.

There is a great potential for mold if you live near a river or in a low-lying area like New Orleans. If you have a damp basement or there is a water leak elsewhere, there is potential for mold spores to be in the air inside the house.

OUTSIDE THE HOUSE

If your home is completely shaded by trees and shrubs, then you know it dries out slowly after wet weather. Some relief may occur if you do some adjustments to the landscaping. Dense bushes and other plants around the foundation often promote dampness. If you have evergreens or other trees and shrubs growing close to the house, cut them back. Be sure branches do not touch the house. Leave an 18-inch space between foliage and the siding of the house. Remove leaves from gutters and around the foundation. Promote ground-water drainage away from the house.

In the winter, condensation on cold outer walls encourages mold growth, but even thick insulation can be invaded if vapor barriers in exterior walls are not effective. Look for such leaks.

INSIDE THE HOUSE

Indoor mold has to be really profuse for these to induce a chronic allergy reaction. The only real clinical problems come from wet basements and leaks in the walls of the house.

Molds will grow if there is sufficient dampness and anything organic, like food.

They grow readily indoors in garbage bins, food storage areas, in wallpaper, on shower curtains, or in any place affected by standing water. Bathroom tiles are not a big problem because the water from the shower washes away the spores.

Molds thrive on humidity (especially greater than 50%) and are difficult to get out of your home unless you lower the humidity. All rooms, especially basements, bathrooms, and kitchens, need ventilation and consistent cleaning with dilute bleach to deter mold and mildew growth.

Usually, indoor molds and mildew are easily eliminated once you discover them unless you have a leak. Dampness is the single most important factor in mold growth, and it's not always easy to get rid of, especially damp basements and leaks.

SOME MOLD BUSTERS

- First see an allergy specialist to determine if you are allergic to mold. There is no point spending large sums of money if mold allergy is not the reason for your symptoms.

- Get the facts. For a precise measure of the humidity in your home, pick up a humidity gauge at almost any hardware store.

- Keep humidity below 50 percent throughout your house by using a dehumidifier or central or window air conditioner. (Make sure you change the filters regularly so you don't create a situation to increase mold.)

- Keep the basement dry. This is the major source of indoor mold.

- Exhaust the bathroom. A bathroom gets damp and will remain so unless it is well ventilated. A good way to discourage mold is to install an exhaust fan, if not in the ceiling, then in a window. Check the bathroom for leaks. You may need to regrout or recaulk to be sure water isn't seeping under the tiles or tub. Molds thrive in the tiles and grout, and on the inside of the shower curtain. A good scrubbing is better than using fungicides and other chemical cleaners. But mold can sometimes be wiped away using chlorine bleach and water (one ounce to one quart) or another fungicide. Clorox, Tilex, Lysol, and Zephiran chloride are good fungicides. Also, remove bathroom carpeting.

- Damp windowsills and frames are attractive to molds.

- If mold or mildew is visible in carpeting and

wallpaper, remove these items from the house. Never put carpeting on concrete or damp floors because it encourages mold (and dust mites).

- In addition to the basement, don't forget to check humidity in out of the way spots, such as a crawl space, attic, closets, or laundry room.

- Storing firewood in the house imports mold and increases humidity. Wood gives off a surprising amount of moisture as it dries out.

- Wrapping cold-water pipes in insulation will prevent them from sweating and decrease dampness in such closed-in areas.

- Promptly repair and seal leaking roofs or pipes.

- Add fungicides to paint, primer, or wallpaper paste to slow fungus growth on treated areas. This will have little effect if excess moisture remains.

- Don't use foam rubber and polyurethane bedding or pillows or furnishings because they are especially prone to mold invasion.

- Throw away or recycle old books, newspapers, clothing, and bedding.

- Check bookcases for mold growth. In a damp environment mold spores love to settle into books.

- Clean garbage pails frequently.

- Clean refrigerator door gaskets.

IF YOU BUY A DEHUMIDIFIER

Dehumidification can be done via an air conditioner in hot weather, or with a special dehumidifier machine in any weather.

Correct venting and fans can also be helpful. For example, an exhaust fan is a useful tool against localized humidity in a bathroom or laundry room. A fan and vent in an attic or a room with a very high ceiling can clear heat and humidity from a fairly large area.

Using a dehumidifier in a damp basement may be helpful, but in general it cannot control humidity throughout the house. Empty the water in the dehumidifier and clean units regularly to prevent mold from growing.

If you buy a dehumidifier, use a reliable retailer, who will take the time to help you determine what size machine(s) you need for your situation. From the physician's point of view, the most important thing about a machine is that it be kept clean—clean it daily—or the mold will proliferate in the tank and cause you more problems. You can actually smell mold flourishing in some dehumidifiers. Follow the cleaning directions scrupulously. The machine should come with a solution that will prevent mold growth.

A dehumidifier is an appliance that is available for as little as $200 and more than $1,000. Some are equipped with a high-efficiency pump for removing condensation that has collected in the bucket. A long hose attaches to drain water from the unit to any location above the unit. It has an automatic shut off and antibacterial filter. If you go for the top of the line, you can buy a portable air conditioner and dehumidifier combination. This machine can be wheeled anywhere, giving you cool comfort when you need it. It's ideal for use where window and central air-conditioning is not feasible in your home or office. Both units function as a dehumidifier, can be quickly vented with a hose for portable use, or can be installed for regular use. Some models cool up to 250 square feet.

The most important consideration is the size. A cheap model is not likely to remove much humidity, unless it is in a very small room. To be effective in a basement, you need a much larger unit. If you have a newer house you may be able to install a central dehumidification system. If you are building a new home in a damp area, consider adding this feature.

GET SOME PROFESSIONAL ADVICE

If you know you are allergic to mold—were tested by an allergist, and believe your home is harboring mold that you may not be aware of—consider hiring professional cleaners or exterminators to eliminate mold growth throughout your home.

Or, if you do the job yourself, a good source of information is the U.S. Government Printing Office,

Superintendent of Documents, Washington, DC 20402. Write for their free pamphlet, "How to Prevent and Remove Mildew."

Toxic Molds Are Not Allergens

Some molds found indoors may produce toxins that cause health problems, but this is not an allergic response. We don't know much about toxic molds, but we are learning. We do know about the stachybotrys mold that tends to flourish in the wake of floods or heavy rains. It can be found in plaster board walls, among other places. When wet it appears black and slimy, and when it is dry it looks dusty.

This mold may cause illness. Symptoms may include headaches, muscle aches, fatigue, respiratory problems, and rashes.

In 1997, an historic library in Staten Island, New York (a typically damp region) had to be closed because the stachybotrys had infested the ventilation system and walls. In 1994 in Cleveland, a low-lying city on the shore of Lake Erie where many neighborhoods had been afflicted with flooding, an outbreak of lung bleeding in babies was associated with exposure to this mold. While it is rare, this mold is nevertheless potentially dangerous. If you live in a home that has been flooded, throw out or dry out damp materials as soon as possible. If you have unusual symptoms, see your doctor.

FOOD MOLD IS NOT AN ALLERGEN

There is no cross-reaction between allergy to airborne molds and "moldy" foods such as mushrooms, dried fruit, vinegar, or foods with yeast. These can be eaten by anyone with allergy to mold.

"Fermented" wines, especially red wine, may cause nasal congestion for other reasons, especially as wines often contain the chemical histamine. This, however, has nothing to do with allergy to mold.

ALLERGY CHECKLIST

✓ Mold thrives in dead leaves so fall is a particularly "allergic" time.

✓ Grain-growing states in the Midwest have a seasonal mold problem.

✓ There are ways to test for indoor mold to confirm your allergy.

✓ Most allergies are generally from exposure to outdoor molds.

✓ Indoor molds are primarily in basements and leaky walls.

✓ Lowering the humidity will get rid of mold.

✓ A dehumidifier will not do much good unless it is big enough.

✓ Toxic molds are not allergens.

5

DUST MITES:
THE PERENNIAL SCOURGE

Dust mites are to year-round allergies what ragweed is to seasonal allergies. They are king. Perennial allergy symptoms are primarily from airborne allergens found in homes with dust mites. And it's not the critters themselves that cause the problem, but what they produce. The allergen is in the secretions of the unwelcome bugs. A potent allergen in the fecal matter of dust mites, for example, not dust itself, is what makes you sneeze. They live on human dander—that's your skin. Roach droppings also produce lots of allergens, but at least you can see them to get rid of them. Mites are invisible to the naked eye, but if you've ever seen a picture of one magnified under a microscope, it is definitely a creepy crawler. Millions may live in your pillow and you will never want to lie down again.

Scientists don't know why yet, but dust mites

seem to be on the rise. One theory is that it may be due to the tighter housing construction that leaves less ventilation and makes homes more humid. Or it may be the popularity of wall-to-wall carpeting in new homes or the preference for cold water washing, which fails to kill dust mites in bedding and clothing.

SEPARATING DUST MITES FROM DUST

Ordinary house dust may make you sneeze, but the dust itself is not the allergen. It only aggravates your sensitive nasal passages. And those dust bunnies in the corner are usually not the problem either, unless they harbor dust mites or pet allergens to which you are allergic.

There are so many ingredients in "house dust" that it took scientists quite some time to figure out it wasn't the dust itself but what the dust was composed of that was causing allergic symptoms. House dust may include mold, dust mites and their fecal

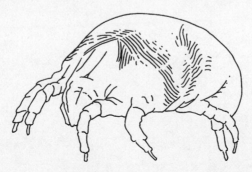

Dust Mite (Illustration is greatly enlarged.)

matter, animal hair and dander, breakdown products of upholstery, lint, and other fibers. It may also contain flakes of human skin, bits of plants, food remnants, cockroach fragments, and much more.

A Dutch scientist in 1920 claimed that dust mites were an allergen but his research was ignored. Later, a German researcher discovered that mites live on human dander. His advice was also ignored until the 1960s and 1970s, when yet another Dutch scientist and a Japanese researcher each established the dust mite's worldwide role in causing allergy. By the 1980s, researchers narrowed it down to the fecal matter from the dust mites that was the allergen. Each dust mite produces about 20 of these microscopic waste particles every day, and more than 100,000 mites may be in your pillow, mattress, or carpet. About 7,000 of them can fit on a dime. Female dust mites put out about 50 eggs at a time. They produce a new generation every three weeks.

These microscopic insects are from the spider, tick, and flea family and are found indoors in most parts of the world. In the northeastern and southeastern United States, about 99 percent of homes are havens for them because they find adequate heat and humidity.

The highest levels are found when the humidity is above 50 percent. Like mold spores, dust mites cannot live in very dry environments. If you live in Denver, you may be safe from mites because it's high up and therefore dry. Mites generally cannot live in altitudes higher than 5,000 feet—unless the homes are humidified.

Banishing the Skin Eaters

There are many species of dust mites, but the ones that concern us are known as the skin eaters. Your body is constantly shedding skin, and this shedding adds to the general dust around you. Shed human skin offers a high-protein diet—and the mites hang out in environments where there's lots of it, such as bedding, upholstery, and carpeting. The fecal matter of the dust mite is a potent protein. This is what you inhale all night long from an old pillow. When the mites' feces land on a mucous membrane, it takes only 30 seconds for your allergy symptoms to begin. You may have a swollen congested nose in the morning from lying down on the mites in your pillows all night.

Before you begin your campaign against mites, make sure they exist—and that you are indeed allergic. The best approach is to see your doctor and get tested. Allergy specialists do this by skin testing, but general physicians can also check for dust-mite allergy by a blood RAST test (see chapter 7).

If you are allergic you should buy a humidity gauge in your hardware store or home center. Try to control the humidity to keep it below 40 percent. (See chapter 4.) Higher than that will invite the mites to make a home with you. Mites generally thrive at humidity in excess of 50 percent.

One woman went to great expense to buy allergen-proof covers for her bedding, and redo her bedroom floors, but her symptoms continued. It turned out she was not allergic to dust mites, but to pollen that was blowing in her bedroom window.

BEGIN WITH A NEW PILLOW

Dust mites love to sleep in your bed. It's full of cozy places where they can congregate and multiply. They live in feather as well as synthetic pillows and comforters. And by the way, hypoallergenic bedding is not going to make a difference in your symptoms. The term hypoallergenic only means the product is made with materials that do not themselves cause allergy. Stuffed material of any type will support dust mite growth and allow accumulation of dust mite allergen.

Getting rid of a pillow full of dust mites is the single most important factor to controlling your allergy to dust mites. Some people never throw away pillows. In fact, some pass them down for generations— especially down pillows, which people often consider too expensive or valuable to throw away. One woman had pillows from her great-grandmother's home in Europe, where these pillows were made with eiderdown, the small breast feathers from ducks. (In this country goose feathers are used.) So she treasured her pillows—and suffered.

Treat yourself to a new pillow and then cover it with a special allergen-proof zipped casing. These are no longer just made of plastic, but from very breathable fabrics that are just like good cotton. If you don't encase the pillow with this protection, after six months your new pillow will be infested again. If you don't get a new pillow, then covering your old one with the special allergy covers may be adequate.

STOP SLEEPING WITH THE ENEMY

Studies show that if you minimize dust mite exposure in your bedroom your allergic symptoms will decrease and you'll need less medication. Encasing your bedding—pillows, mattress, box spring—is therefore considered one of the primary steps in reducing your allergy symptoms. Comforters and duvets should also be covered with allergy-proof airtight material. Make sure you buy these coverings from reputable allergy supply sources. (See Appendix B for a list.)

Wash these casings and your bedsheets weekly in very hot water. To kill the mites you must wash at temperatures of at least 130 degrees. Most cities have laws that limit the temperature of hot water to 125° to avoid scalding children. A hot dryer may also help to kill dust mites.

BARE YOUR FLOORS

Get rid of wall-to-wall carpeting in the bedroom, because mites sink into the pile and you can't get them out. Also, if the carpet is laid on a concrete floor, humidity may be trapped and this will increase the number of dust mites.

No vacuum can significantly reduce the number of mites in your carpet, even with short pile carpeting. Many vacuums are now advertised with HEPA filters to trap tiny dust mite particles (see chapter 12). Steam cleaning only adds moisture to the mite environment. It may even contribute to their growth.

Several products, such as Dustmitex, are available to reduce mite growth in carpets, but it is still unclear how much they help.

Hardwood, tile, or linoleum is better for you, because you can damp mop such floors regularly to control dust. If you must have a rug, use a washable or dry-cleanable throw rug with low pile. An Australian study showed that if you put small rugs in the hot sun, the heat will force the mites to leave after a time as it is too hot. Be sure to take the rugs inside before dark, when it gets cool, or the mites will return.

OTHER UPHOLSTERED PLACES

Other parts of your home need your attention, too, especially places like the couch or easy chairs where you spend lots of time. If your family spends many hours in front of the TV, they are shedding lots of skin to attract dust mites.

High humidity, foam rubber upholstery, and carpeting will encourage mites, so if you or anyone in your family is allergic to dust mites, think about slipcovers that can be frequently washed, or plastic or leather upholstery. Vacuum frequently with a HEPA filter. (See chapter 12 for housekeeping hints to keep dust mites down.)

Think of all the shed skin—and thus, dust mites—that accumulates in movie theater seats. Thousands of people inhabit these places every day, so there may be more shed skin than in your home. Four hours for a concert or play is plenty of time for the dust mites to get to you. Try to attend such functions in theaters with good air-conditioning systems. If necessary, take your medications before you go. The good news is you don't spend much time there, so you can take precautions first. (See chapter 8 on medications.)

MAKE THE CAR CAREFREE

Your car is another potential source of allergens if it is carpeted and upholstered in velour or similar fabric. When you buy a car, think leather or plastic interiors. These will be easier to keep clean and free of dust mites.

If you keep your car parked in a damp garage or street, it becomes a haven for mites and mold. (There's also potential for mold in your auto air-conditioning system, in case you are allergic to that.) Turn on the car's air conditioner in damp weather.

Bigger Bad Bugs: Cockroaches

If you live in a multifamily apartment building, even a well-maintained building, you won't be able to avoid the occasional cockroach. Cockroaches have been associated with allergy and asthma in all parts of the world.

It is estimated that more than 10 million Americans are allergic to cockroaches. According to a study reported to the American Academy of Allergy, Asthma and Immunology (AAAAI) in 2001, the prevalence of cockroach allergy ranges from 17 to 41 percent in the United States, and it involves both children and adults. Allergy and asthma are the most common diseases attributable to infestation of cockroaches in housing and is considered a public health concern. While multiple dwellings in cities account for this problem, it occurs whenever substandard housing allows for infestation. This includes rural and semirural areas, as well as suburbs in towns and cities across the country.

About half of inner city allergy patients react positively to skin tests for cockroach sensitivity. If these people inhale cockroach allergen in a bronchial challenge test, they are likely to develop an asthmatic reaction. Allergy to cockroach is considered one of the major causes of the increase in childhood asthma in poor urban areas. While dust mites affect everybody, roach dander is found more often in lower socioeconomic populations.

Cockroach eggs and waste products, as well as the powdery residue of their decomposing bodies, all contribute to allergies, but it's a protein in the cockroach droppings that is the primary trigger of allergy symptoms. When this is inhaled by an allergic person, it can result in allergic rhinitis or, in susceptible patients, to asthma. There's been a lot of concern and publicity about airborne roach matter with children and asthma, but it also causes allergic rhinitis.

Naturally, the best treatment is to avoid them. You can also ask your doctor to test you for allergy to cockroach. Recently, this test has been standardized. (See chapter 7.)

WAYS TO KEEP ROACHES OUT

Even if you are not allergic to them, you don't want cockroaches around, but if you test positive for cockroach allergy, you *must* get rid of them. No one wants them around, but it can be difficult to eliminate them altogether if you live in a multifamily building. Well-maintained buildings usually provide monthly exterminating service, but not all buildings do as good a job. And some families may not want the potent bug poison around, especially if they have pets and small children.

Roaches feel less welcome in a clean, dry house. However, if you see living roaches in your home, try some over-the-counter antiroach products. If this doesn't work, get a professional exterminator and keep the problem under control.

Cockroaches need water to survive and they thrive in high humidity, so make sure to fix and seal all leaky faucets and pipes. (See chapter 3 about lowering the humidity.) You can seal up gaps around pipes and radiators with plain steel wool.

If you don't want to use toxic pesticides, boric acid is effective if it is used properly, although the chalky powder will always be visible. Hardware stores sell boric acid in plastic jars with nozzles on top so you can squirt the powder around the edges of rooms and around plumbing fixtures.

Block areas where roaches could enter your home, including crevices, wall cracks, windows, woodwork or floor gaps, cellar and outside doors, and drains. They often travel through gaps around heat and plumbing pipes.

- To keep roaches from returning, keep food in tight-lidded containers and put pet food dishes away after pets are done eating. Vacuum and sweep the floor after meals.
- Take out garbage and recyclables frequently. Make sure to empty liquid from bottles and dry them.

- Use lidded garbage containers in the kitchen.
- Don't leave used dishes around, especially overnight.
- Clean under stoves, refrigerators, or toasters where loose crumbs can accumulate.
- Another favorite hiding and breeding place is in the folds of the rubber gasket around the refrigerator door.
- Wipe off the stove top and clean other kitchen surfaces and cupboards regularly.
- Make sure you don't bring roaches home in paper bags, boxes, and other packages. Don't collect paper grocery bags or cardboard boxes.
- Accumulated newspapers, paper bags, and boxes are often breeding places for roaches.

ALLERGY CHECKLIST

✓ Dust mites are a major cause of perennial allergies.

✓ Dust mites can't survive in hot, dry environments, or at high altitudes.

✓ Dust mites feed on human dander, the skin you shed.

✓ Encase all your bedding in allergy-proof covers. This is the single best thing you can do to alleviate symptoms.

✓ Getting a new pillow is also very helpful.

✓ Wash bed covers and sheets weekly in very hot water.

✓ Roaches survive anywhere and their droppings are an increasing cause of allergy.

✓ Try commercial remedies to get rid of roaches. If this doesn't work, get professional help from an exterminator.

6

CATS AND DOGS AND OTHER FURRY CRITTERS

Allergy doctors constantly see a spouse or significant other dragging a cat owner (kicking and screaming) to the doctor's office to get treated for allergies. Often, the significant other is developing allergy symptoms from living with the cat and the cat owner. Cat owners themselves are generally in complete denial about the other person's being allergic. The fact that they come in for a visit with an allergist means that a significant other is giving them an ultimatum. This happens generally in a new relationship. If you are allergic to cats, before you accept a date with anyone, ask if they have a cat. If so, then end it right there and save yourself lots of misery. Just convince yourself that you are not attracted to certain types, like blondes or cat owners, for example.

Spouses and significant others are always secondary to the cats. And the cat owners make their families suffer. Children who develop allergies can't come to visit without being overwhelmed with symptoms.

Of the estimated 6 million people who are allergic to cats, one third of them have cats in their homes. Thus, they continue to suffer. If you are allergic to dogs or cats you should not be living with them. This is the cause of much grief, denial, and misery with allergic people. They will do anything to keep their pets. This makes a doctor's job frustrating. People may give up pillows and even dogs, but they will never give up their cats.

Early on with cat patients, the allergy doctor gives them the usual fire-and-brimstone lecture on how they can't get better if they don't give up the cat. It doesn't faze them. The doctor's success rate is close to zero. Success usually comes only when a cat finally dies.

If you are genetically prone to allergies—that is, your family has a personal history of other allergies—it's best to avoid having any pets because your chance of developing allergy is higher and, once bonding with a pet occurs, you will never part with it.

It's Not the Dander or the Fur

The fur may fly from a cat or dog, but the fur itself is not what makes you sneeze and wheeze. Nor is it the dander, although that term is most commonly used in reference to animal allergies.

When a dog or cat makes you sneeze, or your

eyes tear, your immune system is responding to the tiny airborne flakes of dried secretions from skin, saliva, and urine. The hair is inert; your immune system cannot react to hair. However, the hair is a problem because it is coated with saliva or skin secretions or urine. (Think of how often a cat licks itself.) As the animal walks around, microscopic particles of dried saliva break off the hair and become airborne like dust particles. Animal hairs settle to the floor and form fuzz balls with all the other ingredients of dust, but the tiny flakes of protein allergens stay in the air for a long time. If a smell receptor in your nose detects cat urine from the litter box, the allergy receptor in your nose will also detect it and go into action.

Animal allergen is invisible and can land in the lining of your eyes or nose, or be inhaled directly into your lungs. Symptoms usually occur within a few minutes, but in some people symptoms build and become more severe 8 hours after they have had contact with the animal.

Don't think that if the cat or dog is in another room, you won't be exposed to dander. The air and furniture will be full of the animal protein. And if a cat or dog visits your animal-free home, the air in your home is contaminated within 30 minutes.

Airborne animal protein remains on every surface—vertical or horizontal—in your home. If you have carpeting, dander sinks down into the pile. You may succeed only in stirring up trouble rather than ridding the rugs of the dander when you vacuum. Unless it has a special filter, the vacuum will blow the tiny particles right back into the air. (See chapter 12 for ways to lighten the load of allergens in your indoor air.) Regular vacuuming is not effective in decreasing dander because it does not clean the lower levels of carpets and stirs up cat allergen material on top of the carpet, making it airborne.

It can take weeks or months for fabrics to come clean of allergens, and animal allergens may persist for six months or more after the animal has been removed. Fabric, carpet, and clothing can retain cat protein for at least six months. Professional cleaning will help decrease this level substantially.

Most cat owners don't know or understand that the air in their homes is "contaminated" from the cat. They are sure that putting the animal in another room solves the problem. They generally don't understand—and are not sympathetic—when sensitive visitors develop symptoms when the cat is not physically present in the room.

MALE CATS ARE WORSE

More people are allergic to cats than to dogs, and this may be because cats lick themselves more and use a litter box inside the house. All cats are capable of triggering symptoms, but several interesting studies show that male cats produce more allergy protein than females. This amount decreases within a month after the male cats are castrated, so allergen production is under hormonal control.

Is a black cat bad luck for allergy sufferers? According to a January 2000 report in the *Journal of Allergy and Clinical Immunology*, cats with dark coats may provoke more allergic reactions and symptoms than those with lighter colored coats. So far, there has been only one study on this. Researchers at Long Island College Hospital in Brooklyn studied a group of 60 cat owners, most of whom had symptoms of cat allergy. Those with moderate symptoms were more likely to own dark-colored cats than those with mild symptoms. The odds were six times higher with a dark cat. Perhaps dark cats have higher concentrations of antigens, the proteins that prompt the reactions. Or the antigens may be more potent.

CAT ALLERGY WITHOUT A CAT

Even if you don't have a cat, studies show that you can develop allergy to cats simply by being around people who live with cats. That's how pervasive the cat allergen is. It remains airborne if it is undisturbed for long periods of time. In fact, a 1990 study at the University of Virginia found that this might be why your allergic symptoms can come on so quickly if you enter a house with a cat. The reaction is much quicker than your reaction to dust mites would be in the same house. This passive transfer of cat allergen from one environment to another is probably because the allergen is very sticky. Unlike dust mite allergens, animal allergens can stick to things. This is why they are found in such high levels on walls and other surfaces within homes.

But one of the most interesting findings is that you don't even need to live with a cat to develop an allergy and allergic symptoms. You can be exposed in other places. Studies in New Zealand and Australia discovered that children from homes with cats carried the allergen on their clothing to school. Wool and polyester carried higher levels of the allergen than did cotton. For some reason, girls' clothing carried more allergen than did boys'.

In New Zealand there seem to be many homes with cats. The study found that 63 percent of 12-year-old children in that country lived with a cat compared with only 29 percent in Wales, and 42 percent in South Africa.

Investigators believe that because children are exposed to the indoor school environment for so many hours at a time, exposure to high levels of cat allergen can be an important factor for the development of allergic rhinitis and asthma among schoolchildren. Because of this, the investigators believe that carpeting should be discouraged in schools and daycare centers because they may absorb the allergens.

A 1992 Swedish study concluded that the amount of major cat and dog allergens in the dust from

Swedish schools was high enough to induce perennial symptoms in most children with allergy to cats and dogs. More than 50 percent of schoolchildren in that country reported having furry pets at home. The investigators found that the levels of allergens were much higher on chairs than on floors, so they theorize that the allergen is brought in on the clothing of students and teachers. They also concluded that the levels of allergens found were high enough to sensitize children or induce asthma in those already allergic to cats or dogs.

In the United States, the Department of Pediatrics at Johns Hopkins University School of Medicine measured airborne concentrations of cat allergen in homes that had cats and those that did not. This 1995 study found a low level of cat allergen in homes without cats. The investigators theorized that this low level may be capable of inducing symptoms in an allergic person. According to their published report, these researchers found cat allergen "in settled dust samples from homes without cats, as well as in every other building where it has been sought, including newly built homes, shopping malls, doctors' offices, and even hospitals."

Now, how many people in your apartment building own cats?

If You Won't Give Up Your Pet

Many allergists won't treat patients unless they give up their cats, but in reality, most patients won't give them up. Doctors do recognize the psychological importance of having pets. Many medications are available for allergic rhinitis and conjunctivis from pet allergy, but it is important to stay focused on attempting to find another home for the pet. If all else fails, immunotherapy (allergy shots) can be given, which is usually effective (see chapter 9). It is a much more serious problem if you get asthma symptoms as a result of the allergy.

KEEP THE PET OUT OF THE BEDROOM

At least half of the cat owners say their cats sleep with them. One significant other complained that the two cats slept on either side of his girl-friend's head. If you have a cat you must get it out of the bedroom at night. This has about a 30 percent success rate. One woman who did this came in with dark circles under her eyes. The cat spent all night scratching at her door, she said, and she could not sleep. If people are educated long enough, they may eventually part with their cats. The best solution is to find a close friend or family member who will take the pet, so the allergic person can still visit it.

KEEP THE LITTER BOX FAR AWAY

The cat's litter box is a potent source of allergen. If it is not cleaned frequently, and you can smell it, this can set off your allergic response mechanisms. For this reason, it is a good idea to keep it in a room of the house that is as far away as possible from the main activity rooms. Especially, make sure it is far from your bedroom. Also, change the box often—and get somebody else to do that chore, if possible.

GIVE YOUR CAT A BATH—VERY CAREFULLY

Some studies have shown that bathing dogs and cats on a weekly basis may reduce the amount of allergy material that is shed in the home for approximately the two following days each time the pet is washed. It's unclear, however, how much this really helps. Ideally you must soak the cat briefly in a sink full of water; soap is not necessary. Not many cats will tolerate a bath, so you may risk more physical harm to yourself from the cat's resistance. (Wiping the pet with a damp cloth is usually not enough; they need to be dunked in the water because the allergens are on the skin.)

If you work away from home during the week, it might be some help if you give your cat a Friday evening bath. That way, you can reduce the amount of allergen in the air over the weekend.

One allergist, who realized his patient was never

going to part with the cat, suggested a cat bath once a week. The next time the patient came into the office, she was covered with bandages and bruises. He thought she had been in a car accident.

"It's your fault," the irate patient told him. "You suggested the bath."

ONCE THE CAT HAS GONE

If you are one of the few allergic cat owners who decides to part with your furry pet, the allergen will not leave the air in your home overnight. Cat allergen will persist in the air inside your home for as long as six months. And, assuming your cat slept with you, the allergen will be in your mattress for long after the cat leaves. You may need new bedding, but at least you should encase the mattress, box spring, and pillows with impermeable covers mentioned in chapter 5 about dust mite allergy. You can speed up the air cleansing by extensive use of environmental controls such as removing carpets and upholstered furniture.

The Hairless Dog Theory

Dogs are also a major cause of pet allergy. As with cats, the allergen is in the dog's saliva, secretions from skin glands, and urine. Because dogs lick themselves less than cats and tend to urinate outdoors, dog allergy is somewhat less of a problem than cat allergy.

There are no hypoallergenic breeds of dog or cat. The old theory was that dander stuck to animal hair, so if the pet did not shed hair, no dander would get into the air. A week with a poodle may convince you this is true, but if you are sensitive, the allergy will develop over time. Poodles, bichon frises, Portuguese water dogs, and terriers all were thought not to shed and thus made acceptable pets for the allergic. Stories of having a poodle and not reacting are legion but are mostly individual incidents that can be explained. Either the person was not very allergic to begin with, the animal spent most of its time outdoors or lived in a house with no upholstery or carpets, or there was an air-cleaning machine.

A cat or dog produces a certain amount of allergen per week, and this amount can vary from animal to animal, but all breeds are capable of triggering symptoms. If you are sensitive enough, you can have a reaction in a public place from dander that has been transported on a pet owner's clothing.

Little Rodents, Big Allergens

Small as they are, rabbits, hamsters, guinea pigs, and other rodents cause as much if not more trouble than a cat or dog. Rodents kick up dust. (Think of that hamster racing around on his exercise wheel in his case.) Parents who offer to take home the school pet for summer vacation often report problems with allergies. These animals are usually hamsters, gerbils, or rabbits. Once school is closed and the animal is living in your house, it's hard to find another parent to take on this chore.

Urine is the prime source of allergens. Rodent urine is high in protein and it is often sprayed rather than deposited. This creates greater exposure to the air. After urine dries, proteins become airborne and are inhaled. And like the mouse's archenemy, the cat, it is the male that produces the most allergen—four times as much as the female.

If you have mice in your home, they can spew a surprisingly large amount of their allergen into the air. A woman who had suffered mild allergy symptoms suddenly became chronically symptomatic when she moved into a brand new home in the suburbs. She could not figure out the cause. The family had no pets, the house wasn't moldy, but it was inside the house that she suffered constant sneezing and runny nose and eyes. Eventually, she discovered that field mice were entering the house through a faulty dishwasher installation. An allergy test confirmed the fact that she was indeed allergic to rodents. The entry into the house for the mice was blocked and the woman's symptoms ceased.

If you live in a building where there may be rodents, be sure to have it professionally exterminated. Ironically, having a cat would keep the mice away, but if you are allergic to cats, too, it would only make your life worse.

Birds of a Feather

A woman who lived in a two-story house told her doctor that she wheezed when she walked down the stairs from her bedroom, but never when she walked up the stairs. This seemed odd, since the effort of going up would tend to be more strenuous. However, she felt better within an hour after being downstairs. The doctor could not figure out what was wrong. He had asked her the usual questions, about whether there was anything in the house she could possibly be allergic to. She said no. She didn't appear to have any allergies. However, one day, she happened to be showing him some pictures of her family, and the doctor asked, "What's that on your shoulder?"

"Oh, that's my parrot," she replied. "And where does it live?" the doctor asked. "He lives in a cage in my bedroom, but I cover the cage at night."

Healthy birds spend lots of time preening, fluffing their feathers, and shaking feathers and debris all over the place. This causes release of feather dust. Birds also molt regularly, some constantly, and others at certain times of the year.

Bird allergen comes from the powdery-like feather dust that collects in and around the bird's case. This dust, especially from cockatoos and cockatiels, builds up rapidly in the room that contains the cage and circulates through the house. Another source of dust is the droppings that have dried in the bottom of the cage. And birds create a good deal of waste. Most birds, experts say, produce from 25 to 50 eliminations a day. Birds are also sloppy and the area all around the cage gets messy quickly.

ISOLATE THE CAGE

If you are allergic to birds but can't part with your pet, take some steps to reduce the amount of allergen you are breathing in. Put the bird in a room you don't spend much time in. Stand the cage on a sheet of plastic that can be taken away and cleaned. To keep feather dust and droppings to a minimum, change the papers in the bottom of the cage at least once a day. Vacuum up all around the cage to get rid of debris and loose feathers. Also, wipe the washable surfaces with a damp sponge. Damp-mop wood floors. Cleaning up with dry clothes and brooms will only send more of the allergens into the air. Another way to keep allergens to a minimum is to have an air purifier in the room.

A BIRD'S BATH

While the cage should be cleaned daily, at least once a month you need to take the bird out and scrub the cage thoroughly with water and bleach. Try to get someone else to do this job. Pet stores sell special bathing cups for birds, and giving your bird a bath or a shower may keep feather dust allergen release down. Pet stores also sell something to spray on the bird to keep feather dust down, but this has not been proven to be effective.

Better yet, put a birdbath on your lawn or garden and watch the wild birds bathe.

Horse Allergy

There hasn't been much study about horse allergy, but we presume a protein from the animal comes in contact with your skin. One woman was fine when she was outside with her horse, but in the barn she began sneezing and wheezing. Another woman was okay when she walked her horse, but when she rode the horse until the horse worked up a lather, she got hives right through her jeans from the horse sweat. Some people only sneeze around the horse, but get hives if the horse saliva touches their skin.

The only way to find out is to get tested.

If you spend time in a barn occupied by a horse or horses, the air will be filled with allergen. A barn also usually contains hay, a source of mold or grass pollen. Some are allergic to the hay. There's lots of pollen mixed up with the hay.

At one time, horsehair was used as stuffing for mattresses and furniture. It is still used in some furniture and mattresses. However, it is now washed and sterilized before it is put into furniture stuffing so the allergen substances should no longer be present. However, if you have some very old furniture that may contain horsehair, consider having it reupholstered if you think it is a source of allergy symptoms.

ALLERGY CHECKLIST

✓ Most allergic cat owners never get rid of their cats.

✓ It's the animal's secretions that become airborne and cause the allergy symptoms—not the dander or hair.

✓ Male cats produce more allergens than female cats.

✓ Animal allergens stick to every horizontal and vertical surface in your home, as well as your clothing.

✓ Cat allergens on other people's clothing can cause you to have allergy symptoms even if you don't live with a cat.

✓ There are no hypoallergenic breeds of cat or dog.

✓ Rodent allergens are very potent.

✓ Pet birds can be a source of airborne allergy.

✓ Horse allergens have not been studied as widely as those of other pets.

PART II

How Your Doctor
Can Help You

7

WHEN YOU NEED AN ALLERGIST

It's the four F words that finally bring people to the doctor to get treatment for their allergy symptoms: they feel fuzzy, full-headed, fatigued, and complain about lack of focus. In other words, they are not functioning optimally. And once again it's usually the spouse or significant other who prompts the visit. The person living with the allergic person is sick of listening to the sneezing and sniffing, the throat clearing, the snoring, and seeing tissues all over the house.

Allergic people put up with their symptoms for years. "Oh, it's not that bad," they say. "It's not all the time. I get used to it." They grin and bear it as each pollen season approaches. Or they live with their stuffy noses, without realizing they are allergic to dust mites and sleeping with millions of them in their pillows.

If this is you, then you have forgotten how it feels to be clear, to breathe freely. You owe it to yourself to find out and to make a pact with your doctor. Take the minimum medication to get to a baseline and see what it's like. When they finally get treatment, at least 90 percent of patients say their doctor was absolutely right. Of course, there are always a few who don't like feeling this good. They are not used to their noses being so clear. The sensation of air passing freely through their noses disturbs them!

How to Find an Allergist

Your primary care physician can prescribe allergy medications for seasonal symptoms, but when your allergies are chronic and overwhelming despite your best efforts at avoiding allergens, then it's time to see an allergist. You may need a more comprehensive program of avoidance and medication—and possibly some tests to determine precisely what you're allergic to, or discover an unsuspected allergy.

An allergist is a doctor of internal medicine or pediatrics who specializes in allergies and the immune system. These doctors have typically had four years of medical school, then internships and residency in internal medicine or pediatrics for three years. After that they do an allergy and immunology fellowship for two more years.

Select a doctor who is board certified to treat allergies, who comes highly recommended, who has a track record of helping others with allergies, and one you feel comfortable to work with over a long period of time, if necessary. Keep in mind, however, that the only long-term care is if you undergo a course of immunotherapy (allergy shots).

Your local medical society can confirm for you that a particular doctor who claims to specialize in treating allergies is in fact board certified. There are also Web sites where you can look up physicians' certification. The American Academy of Allergy, Asthma, and Immunology (AAAAI) can also help you to locate a doctor in your community. (See Appendix A.)

While you should not judge a doctor on personality over skill, there are some basic traits that you do want. For example, if a doctor always rushes you, or doesn't seem terribly interested in your story, then perhaps you should look for someone else. A doctor should certainly be a good listener, and give you undivided attention. After all, you are hiring this doctor, so you should be satisfied with what you are paying for. A doctor may have a great reputation in the media, but if the doctor hasn't the time for you, it's not likely you'll get the individual treatment you deserve. Trust yourself and your feelings about a doctor.

WORKING WITH YOUR DOCTOR

The purpose of allergy treatment is to help you function normally in the world. Some doctors are especially good at teaching their patients to care for themselves; they encourage them to live as fully as possible.

All other things being equal, this is the kind of doctor you want. A good doctor will explain any test to be done and what to expect from medicines prescribed, including side effects. (See chapter 8.) In addition, he or she will do everything possible to give you a sense of self-sufficiency, such as providing literature explaining how to avoid allergens and how to medicate yourself effectively.

A doctor will usually allot more time for your first visit to talk with you about your medical history, and do a physical exam.

The goal of you and your allergist is to determine what is triggering your symptoms and to work to develop a management plan, which includes ways to avoid allergens, and if necessary, using medication or immunology. When a course of treatment is recommended to you, ask what and when results should be expected. The most important service you should expect from your doctor is that you get better as a result of treatment. This seems obvious, but it is sometimes overlooked. If nothing seems to work, consider getting a second opinion from another doctor. Your first doctor may simply have missed something, such as an element of your history that was important.

It is your responsibility to work with your doctor by avoiding allergens as much as possible and taking your medications or treatments as prescribed. Once you are satisfied, then make a commitment to continue treatment as long as you need it, although long-term treatment is needed only when getting allergy shots.

Once the doctor has given you an estimate of what your treatment is likely to include and cost, you can then turn to your insurance company to find out what's covered and also if the doctor's fees are within the normal range.

TELLING YOUR ALLERGY STORY

Your history is the major tool in diagnosis, so when you first visit an allergist, do some homework ahead of time. In addition to telling about your own medical history, you should know what major illnesses affected close relatives, and of course, whether anyone in your family has allergies— defined as any of these:

- Hay fever
- Asthma
- Eczema
- Food, drug, or bee sting reactions
- Hives

Talk with your relatives. You'll be surprised at how often people are unaware of family medical history. In the past, few people talked about illnesses or conditions. It was not considered cool. It is only in recent decades that we are so much more health conscious. But others may recall that your paternal grandmother always sneezed around the cats. Perhaps one of your parents always had "lots of colds" in the fall, or runny eyes whenever they went on camping trips, but the condition was never diagnosed as allergies. If you have children or a child is coming for treatment, be sure you know as much about your spouse's history, too.

Also bring a list of the medications you take regularly including aspirin and prescription drugs—or bring the drugs with you. Naturally, if you had previous treatment for allergies, especially allergy tests, then bring those records.

In telling your story, a doctor will lead you to information he or she needs to determine that you indeed have allergies—or if some symptoms may be caused by something else.

What is your chief complaint? Narrow the problem to the most troublesome feature: runny nose, itching in your ears, burning eyes. Be ready for detailed follow-up questions from the doctor. If you have a cough, you will be asked whether you cough up mucus and if so, what color it is and other questions about it. If you have ear pain, you will be asked whether you have run a fever in connection with it.

Describe your symptoms. Think about your symptoms and better yet, write them down before your visit so you don't forget them. How often do they occur, when, and where? When did the symptoms first appear? If possible give an exact date. At least try to give the time of year and how many months or years ago these symptoms began. Many people have had allergies so long before they get help that they can't recall when they began.

Your allergist will ask questions like these:

- Are your symptoms year-round or seasonal?
- Do they change with location: geography, urban or suburban or rural areas, or from being inside to going outside?
- Do they worsen with exposures to cats or other animals?
- What are the triggers and exacerbating factors?
- Have you had any previous evaluations for your symptoms?
- What, if any, treatment has been tried so far?

Be honest about your environment, too. Some people think if they don't mention they have a pet, the allergist won't find out and they can just get some medication and the allergy will go away. (Remember those cat people. And the lady with the parrot who didn't think the bird played a role in her allergies.) You need to tell the doctor about the pets, and how long you've had them. Also describe your home environment. Is it dry or damp? It's important

for the allergist to know if you have a damp basement that might be harboring mold.

PHYSICAL EXAMS AND TESTS

A fairly complete physical examination will focus
on your head—ears, eyes, nose, throat, neck—as
well as lungs, heart, abdomen, and skin. An allergist
will look for characteristic signs of allergy as well as
other causes of your symptoms. For example, a pale
gray-blue, boggy lining inside your nose is characteristic of allergic rhinitis. However, a polyp or evidence of infection may point to a nonallergic cause
of the trouble.

Today's sophisticated diagnostic techniques mean
your doctor can get a very clear look at what's going
on in your nose. A flexible endoscope can be inserted
into your nose and record findings on a video screen.
The cells in your nasal fluid can be tested if necessary. And if you have chronic and complicated symptoms that include sinusitis, even a CT scan can be
called for.

Blood tests are generally not necessary if you have
inhaled allergies. Such tests are more helpful for people with severe skin diseases like eczema or systemic
diseases that are allergy related.

Subsequent visits to an allergist will be shorter,
unless you need more in-depth testing.

When You Need Allergy Tests

You don't have to get rid of your cat if you are allergic to dust mites and not cats. And if your allergy is seasonal, you don't need medications all year long. But if you have symptoms even when you are not near the cat, then other allergens are obviously involved.

Once you have described your symptoms and the doctor evaluates your history, then almost always a screening series of allergy skin tests is suggested to determine sensitivity. Your allergies can change over the course of your life and should be tested periodically to see if you are still allergic to the same things or new ones.

You should be retested periodically because allergies wax and wane. You could lose your allergy to grass pollen, but develop one to dust mites. If you lived in Chicago and ragweed gave you symptoms, they may come from sagebrush if you move to the Southwest.

The purpose of allergy tests is to:

- confirm allergy diagnosis
- differentiate from other disorders
- discover unsuspected allergy
- guide treatment

Adults and children of any age can be tested for allergies.

Common allergens tested include:

- Dust mites
- Cat, dog, or other furry animal
- Molds in your home or in the air outside
- Tree, grass, and weed pollen
- Cockroach

These are all proteins. The allergen extracts used in allergy tests are made commercially and are standardized according to FDA requirements. In the past 10 to 20 years, standardization has greatly increased, and your allergist is able to safely test you for allergies to substances using these extracts.

Some people only need one test to confirm what they suspect about a specific allergy, such as dust mites, before they go to great expense. Tests take a few minutes and you get results right away. These tests are quick and highly accurate. The number of tests you get is highly variable, depending on your case. The average is 15 to 70, but it varies with different doctors in different parts of the country.

PRICK TESTS

Drops of allergens are placed in a row on your skin—along your back or the inside of your forearm. Each one is pricked with a needle. If you have an allergy, the specific allergens that you are allergic to will set off a reaction. If a reaction occurs—a red bump like a mosquito bite—then you are allergic.

Remember, if you are allergic, you have the IgE antibody, which binds to the allergy substance; this activates mast cells to release chemicals called mediators—such as histamine—that cause redness and swelling. With testing, this swelling occurs only in the spots where the tiny amount of allergen has been scratched onto your skin. So, if you are allergic to ragweed pollen but not to cats, the spot where the ragweed was scratched to your skin will swell and itch a bit, forming a small wheal, usually about the size of a dime. The spot with cat allergen will remain normal.

This reaction happens quickly, within 15 minutes, so you don't have to wait long to find out what is triggering your allergies. In general, you won't have any other symptoms from the test besides the slightly swollen wheal where the test was done. This goes away in a half hour and your skin surface returns to normal. If there is any itching, tell your doctor about it. If you have a severe allergy, you may also experience some of your normal allergy symptoms at the time.

The number of prick tests you get depends on how severe your symptoms are, and how many allergens you are likely to be exposed to given your history and geographic location. As many as 70 tests could be required, but in most cases, this number is never needed.

If you have a history that suggests a severe allergy, your doctor will either test with a much weaker test material first or do a blood RAST (radioallergosorbent) test as a screen (see next section). If there is no reaction to the weak test, then the regular strength can be applied. In extremely rare cases, a severe allergy exists that is not predicted from the history. In such cases, patients may get systemic symptoms, such as shortness of breath, along with a larger skin reaction to the test. You may then require an injection of epinephrine.

If you have severe skin disease such as severe eczema, you won't be able to get skin tests.

Antihistamines or some antidepressants can block your body's histamine and result in a negative test. Thus, you have to stop using them from 48 to 72 hours before testing or it will interfere.

BLOOD (RAST) TEST

Blood tests are generally used only in cases in which skin tests cannot be performed, such as on people with skin conditions, or who are taking medications that would limit the test. It is also used as a first screening for a reaction on people with very severe allergies.

Diagnosis of allergy by a blood test—looking for specific IgE antibody in the blood—can be done either by RAST (radioallergosorbent) or a similar test called ELISA. Drawing blood costs more than skin pricks and the results are not available as rapidly as they are with the skin tests. The blood test is only available for a limited number of allergens. It is as specific but less sensitive than skin testing. This test will detect the specific allergy but may miss a low-level allergy that skin testing will pick up.

INTRADERMAL TEST

If a prick test is negative, but the allergy is still suspected, an allergist may do an intradermal test. This puts the test material between layers of the skin. There is some flexibility this way to try weaker doses of test material and follow with a stronger strength. There are different "top" strengths for prick or intradermal tests. If someone is not positive to a "top" dose, it is very unlikely they have a significant allergy.

ALLERGY CHECKLIST

✓ After years of procrastination, people admit they feel better with medical treatment.

✓ An allergist is a medical doctor who specializes in allergies and the immune system.

✓ You need to work with your doctor to manage your allergy symptoms.

✓ Your history is the major diagnostic tool for the allergist.

✓ It's important to talk with relatives to find out who else in the family had any kind of allergy.

✓ Allergy skin tests are an easy and standardized way to confirm or identify allergies.

✓ Blood tests are used if skin tests cannot be done, but they are less specific than prick tests.

✓ Because allergies change, you need to be retested periodically.

8

THE RIGHT MEDICATION
AT THE RIGHT TIME

If you were a diabetic, you would not wait until you were in a coma to take your insulin. You'd take insulin to prevent such an extreme response, just as you would take your high blood pressure medications to avoid a stroke. But few people with allergies use the same logic. They wait until the symptoms appear—and it takes some suffering to get them under control. People are amazingly stoic about allergies! If you use medications properly and try to avoid allergens, you can also avoid being miserable.

Some people manage their allergies with over-the-counter antihistamines and decongestants. This self-treatment approach may be okay for short-term flare-ups of mild symptoms, but it's best to be under a doctor's care.

If you use over-the-counter decongestant sprays habitually, you only create more problems. These nasal sprays will clear your sinuses and shrink swollen nasal membranes, but if you take them longer than twice a day for three days, they cause rebound congestion. When the drug wears off, swelling in your nose becomes even greater than it was to begin with. Some people will use the spray again and repeat the cycle until their nose is totally blocked when the spray wears off. This is known as rhinitis medicamentosum, or decongestant nasal spray addiction.

There is no magic bullet for treating allergies. Rather, it is a sensible management plan that includes avoiding allergens (the best, and ironically, least followed therapy), using medications properly, and staying healthy.

The Priming Effect

One of the most important things to understand about reducing your allergy symptoms, and thus your misery, is the priming effect. Once you are hit with the first grains of pollen, your immune system is "primed." This means it takes less pollen the next time to set off your symptoms. Your mast cells know that more pollen is coming, so they are primed for the next hit. On day one of pollen season, it may take 100 grains of pollen to trigger allergy symptoms and on day 30, it takes only one. In other words, you have increasing sensitivity.

Let's say mold spores are at high levels because of

prolonged rain. Once you've been hit by that itchy throat, watery eye sensation, you are most susceptible to those symptoms every time the wind blows in something new. Even if you do not normally react to allergens, you may start reacting after a first overwhelming blast like the spring's wave of pollens. Once you're primed to be allergic to something, you have an increased chance of becoming allergic to other things, and regretfully you don't need a full dose to get as much suffering.

It's a good idea to treat allergies aggressively and early because of this priming factor. For example, steroid nasal sprays used early can block this priming. People who understand the priming effect have fewer problems with their allergy symptoms than those who take a scattershot approach to their allergies.

Let's start with the most effective medications for allergic rhinitis.

Nasal Steroid Sprays

Nasal steroid sprays are currently the most effective single maintenance therapy available for perennial or seasonal nasal allergy. In fact, these sprays are effective in controlling the four major symptoms of allergic rhinitis, including sneezing, runny nose, itching, and nasal blockage. They work by decreasing inflammation and preventing the allergic reaction.

The newer nasal steroid sprays, such as Flonase,

Nasonex, and Rhinocort, can generally be used once a day, compared to some of the older sprays (Vancenase, Beconase, Nasacort, Nasalide), which took up to a week to achieve maximum benefits.

Because they are so effective, some people can just use them when they need them. About 80 percent of people taking intranasal corticosteroids say their symptoms clear up whether they use them regularly or as needed. A study by Scott M. Kaszuba, M.D., a researcher with the University of Chicago, in the *Archives of Internal Medicine,* compared leading steroid nasal sprays and antihistamines. People using the nasal sprays got more complete symptom relief and better quality of life than those taking antihistamines regularly.

Allergies cause a one-two punch. First the sneezing, and then when that eases off, the congestion sets in. Antihistamines put a stop to sneezing, but nasal sprays actually seem to help the entire allergic response. Dr. Kaszuba randomly assigned steroid nasal spray or antihistamine pills to 88 people suffering ragweed allergies in the fall—peak season in Chicago. Half used nasal spray and half antihistamine pills as needed for 28 days. Each one kept a diary to record symptoms.

Another study (in 1998) reported that half the participants with severe seasonal allergies needed to take antihistamines and a steroid nasal spray to control symptoms.

These new nasal steroids are best used right before a known allergy season or at least by the first hint. Once you have symptoms, it takes longer to work, especially if the inside of your nose is so swollen that the sprays cannot penetrate into the nasal cavity as well.

Intranasal steroids are absorbed into the lining of the nose through your nasal mucosa. At the prescribed doses, these medications don't get into the blood in any significant amount. This is especially important when selecting therapy for children.

Most of these medications are effective if you use them once a day. The newer ones have not been around long enough for long-term studies, but the older nasal steroid sprays have been tested in chronic-use studies for up to 12 years and have proven safe.

INTRANASAL IPRATROPIUM BROMIDE (ATROVENT)

You can probably get adequate relief with an intranasal steroid with or without an antihistamine. In extreme cases, intranasal ipratropium bromide (Atrovent) nasal spray may be needed as a third agent for severe symptoms. This type of spray is effective in reducing runny nose, but does not treat other nasal symptoms, such as stuffiness or sneezing. Side effects may include nasal dryness and crusting.

Atrovent nasal spray is relatively free of side

effects. However, some people feel too dry after using it. Nosebleeds and sore throat can occur in 5 to 10 percent of people who use it for a long period of time.

This may be prescribed if your nose is constantly and profusely running, although it depends on whether or not the cause is allergy or not, and if it is acute or chronic. Options for treatment could include Atrovent or oral decongestants for the immediate relief of symptoms and steroid spray for the longer term.

INTRANASAL CROMOLYN (NASALCROM)

Intranasal cromolyn is often called a mast cell stabilizer, but we don't really know how it inhibits an allergic response. In addition to its primary action, it also has a mild, anti-inflammatory effect. This spray may be useful for preventing or minimizing allergic symptoms just before a known, predictable exposure. For example, if you are allergic to cat, use cromolyn nose spray 30 to 60 minutes before entering a home with a cat. No significant side effects are associated with this medicine, but if you use it to treat constant rhinitis, then you need to use it four times a day. For this reason, it is not widely recommended to treat chronic allergy.

SIDE EFFECTS

Adverse effects from using nasal sprays are usually limited to nasal irritation and bleeding. Nasal ulcers can occur but are extremely rare. To reduce the chance of ulcer formation, it may be helpful to direct the spray in different angles each time it is used. Make sure your doctor examines the inside of your nose periodically.

Headache and nasal congestion are rare side effects and often fade with continued use. While mild nasal bleeding is also rare, if it occurs, stop using the spray and call your doctor. (These sprays are also useful in the treatment of nasal polyps and in the prevention of their recurrence after surgery.)

If you are using an inhaled steroid to control asthma, then make sure you discuss this with your doctor. There is the possibility of additive effects from the sprays if you also use inhaled steroids for the lungs.

USING NASAL SPRAYS CORRECTLY

Most nasal sprays come in pressurized canisters, and you need to shake them gently before using. Also, clear your nose of any mucus first. Keep your head back when you use the spray. Spray one nostril at a time, while pressing your finger against the other to close off the air. Press down on the canister as you begin to breathe in slowly through your nose. Put the canister nozzle at the inside of your nose and insert by aiming slightly toward the eye area and then squirting. Avoid sneezing or blowing your nose immediately after spraying. Ask your doctor to explain how best to use it. Most prescriptions come with instructions for proper use.

If you are using a pump bottle, follow the same steps but prime the pump first. Tilt your head slightly forward. Squeeze the pump as you begin to breathe in slowly through your nose. These are general directions and may vary, so be sure when you get a prescription, ask your doctor to explain how to use it.

It may take up to two weeks of using a nasal steroid spray to see full results. If your nose hurts or bleeds, stop using the spray for a day or two. Keep medicine in a cool place and away from sunlight.

INTRANASAL CORTICOSTEROIDS

Trade Name	Generic Name
Beconase AQ	Beclomethasone dipropionate
Vancenase AQ 84 mcg	Beclomethasone dipropionate
Rhinocort	Budesonide
Nasarel	Flunisolide
Flonase	Fluticasone propionate
Nasonex	Mometasone furoate monohydrate
Nasacort AQ	Triamcinolone acetonide

Antihistamines

Antihistamines, as the name implies, are designed to combat the effect of histamine release from mast cells. Histamines cause your nose to run and also to clog up. If taken in time, antihistamines are very effective in drying you up, but the big problem with over-the-counter antihistamines is they can make you sleepy. The new prescription drugs are less sedating. Other common side effects of antihistamines include dehydration—especially in dry mouth and eyes. Men with enlarged prostates may have difficulty urinating. Constipation is also a side effect. This is why you need to drink plenty of water.

Antihistamines bind directly to receptors for histamine. When histamine is then released during an allergic reaction, its receptor is already occupied with an antihistamine so the histamine can't induce any reaction. Since histamine can't bind to its normal receptors, the chain of events that causes the allergic reaction is interrupted. *This is why doctors recommend taking antihistamines before your symptoms have appeared.* They only work preventively. They do nothing to treat resulting symptoms. This is a major misconception about antihistamines. If you have been outside in the pollen for hours, your nose is running and your eyes are tearing, and you take an antihistamine when you get home, it won't "undo" any of these symptoms. It will just block further symptoms.

Similarly, if you sleep with a pillow full of dust mites and wake up with a stuffy nose, an antihistamine won't do you any good. You need to take it before you go to sleep. (And get a new pillow!)

Anticipate your need. If you are allergic to ragweed and you know the pollen count is higher than expected, take your antihistamine. Don't wait until the sneezing and weeping begin.

Antihistamines are categorized according to two different kinds of receptors they bind to. These are histamine receptor type one and type two (H1 and H2) that are present on many human tissue sites, including the very important capillaries (H1 predominates) and the lining of the stomach (H2 receptors are important). H1 is the type concerned with allergic rhinitis.

H1 antihistamines block the vascular and neural effects of the H1 receptor. Thus, these drugs reduce sneezing, itching, and to some extent, rhinorrhea (runny nose). However, they have very little effect on nasal congestion, which is mediated by the H2 receptor.

To complicate it further, there are first and second generations of receptors. First generation H1 antihistamines are relatively nonspecific in binding to the H1 receptor. Because these agents can cross the brain/blood barrier, they can make you sleepy. By contrast, second-generation agents are less likely to cross the blood/brain barrier, so they are less sedating than first-generation agents. The "blood/brain" barrier is a fatty layer encasing your brain. While oxygen gets through without a problem and blood vessels are able to penetrate this fatty layer, not all drugs can get through the fat. The old antihistamines used to zip right through. The new drugs are lipophobic—meaning they are phobic about fat. It's too much trouble to get through. Allegra and Claritin are like this, so they don't make you sleepy. Zyrtec can make a small percentage of people slightly sleepy, though some people respond differently. It's like caffeine. Some people can't drink coffee before going to bed because it keeps them awake. Others have no problem. It's the same with Zyrtec.

NONSEDATING AND LIGHTLY SEDATING ANTIHISTAMINES

Seldane (terfenadine) was the first nonsedating antihistamine used in the United States. It was pulled from the market in 1997, after it caused an abnormal heart rhythm in some patients, particularly when combined with other medications, which resulted in a higher blood level of Seldane.

Claritin (loratadine) was introduced in the mid-1990s and did not have this effect. Even in excess doses, it did not produce changes in heart function. Thus, it became the drug of choice at the time. Allegra (fexofenadine), Zyrtec, and Clarinex came later.

Although the new antihistamines don't make you drowsy like the old ones do, they only suppress allergic symptoms, they don't cure the allergies. This is why it is so important to use them as directed by your doctor.

Antihistamines come in tablet, capsule, liquid, or injection form.

You may also develop tolerance to antihistamines. This means that the drug may not work as well to relieve your symptoms after you have been taking it for a long period of time. At this point, your doctor may recommend another class of antihistamines for several months, then switch back to the original if needed.

SIDE EFFECTS

The most notorious side effect of antihistamines is sleepiness, and so the old types are great when you go right to bed, but terrible if you take them in the morning. Not everyone feels sleepy, but sometimes there's mental impairment.

Certain antihistamines can also produce heart palpitations (if combined with decongestants), constipation, dry mouth, and nervousness. It is not wise to take them with alcohol or tranquilizers because they add to the sedation effect of the antihistamine.

This is important to consider if you are at risk for narrow-angle glaucoma, or if you are a man with benign prostatic hyperplasia. Keep in mind that first-generation medications may cause moderate to severe constipation if you take other medications such as calcium channel blockers for high blood pressure.

OVER-THE-COUNTER ANTIHISTAMINES

Trade Name	Generic Name
Dimetapp Allergy	Brompheniramine
Chlor-Trimeton	Chlorpheniramine
Tavist-1	Clemastine
Benadryl	Diphenhydramine

Note that Benadryl is also used to treat skin and nasal allergies and also as a mild sedative to help you sleep. It's also used as a cough suppressant. It's a sustained-release capsule that should be swallowed without chewing or crushing.

PRESCRIPTION ANTIHISTAMINES

Trade Name	Generic Name
Oral Nonsedating Antihistamines	
Allegra capsules	fexofenadine hydrochloride
Claritin tablets	loratadine
Claritin Reditabs	"
Claritin syrup	"
Clarinex tabs	desloratadine
Oral Less-sedating Antihistamines	
Zyrtec tablets	Cetirizine HCl
Zyrtec syrup	"

Trade Name	Generic Name

Oral Non-sedating Antihistamine-decongestant Combinations

Allegra-D	fexofenadine/ pseudoephedrine HCl
Claritin-D 12-hour	Loratadine/ or pseudoephedrine HCl
Claritin-D 24-hour	"
Zyrtec D 12-hour	Cetirizine/ pseudoephedrine

Oral Less-sedating Antihistamine-decongestant Combinations

Semprex-D capsules	Acrivastine/pseudo- ephedrine HCl

Intranasal Antihistamines

Astelin Nasal Spray	Azelastine HCl

Intranasal Mast Cell Stabilizers

Nasalcrom	Cromolyn sodium

Intranasal Anticholinergics

Atrovent Nasal Spray	Ipratropium bromide

Decongestants

Decongestants are often combined with antihistamines to relieve nasal congestion. Decongestants alone, such as Sudafed (pseudoephedrine), do not relieve any other symptom of allergic rhinitis, however, and they have problematic side effects for some people. They stimulate the central nervous system and cause insomnia. Because decongestants shrink the blood vessels to lessen the amount of fluid that leaks out, this can also elevate your blood pressure. There is a wide range of cardiovascular effects including palpitations, arrhythmias, and even hypertensive crises.

They are available in liquid and tablet form both over the counter and by prescription.

Decongestants are also available as a nose spray or in drop form for acute congestion. However, over-the-counter nasal sprays should not be used more than three or four days in a row. As mentioned earlier, prolonged use can cause rebound rhinitis and actually increase your nasal congestion. When the drug wears off, swelling becomes even greater than it was to begin with. Using the spray again and repeating the cycle will eventually cause your nose to become totally blocked when the spray wears off. This is known as rhinitis medicamentosum, or decongestant nasal spray addiction.

Prescription nasal sprays and drops do not have

this effect and can be used for a longer period of
time.

Medications for Treating
Allergic Conjunctivitis

Often when your eyes itch, tear, or swell from allergies, you also have a runny nose and other symptoms of an allergic reaction. Those jittery mast cells
are not only in your nose, but in the membrane covering your eyeballs—the conjuctiva. And these mast
cells act up when airborne allergens get into your
eyes.

EYE DROPS

You can try eye drops alone, but more commonly
you will need antihistamine plus eye drops. And
avoid the pollen as much as possible.

Artificial tears will help to lubricate, dilute, and
remove allergens in your eyes. In some cases, irrigat-
ing your eyes with artificial tears or saline solution
can bring temporary relief. Cold compresses offer
significant relief from eye itching or stinging.

Keep eye medications in the refrigerator. This will
give you additional relief immediately when you put
the cool drops into your eyes.

Not all eye drops are the same, or suited for all
problems. Some treat redness, or dry eyes, or itchiness. If you want to clear up bloodshot eyes that

have been exposed to chlorine, wind, or other irritants, then Clear Eyes, VasoClear, Visine, Nefrine, and OcuClear are good. Prolonged use can cause rebound redness, however.

When your eyes itch because of pollen and other allergens, and oral and nasal allergy medications don't help, then antihistamine eye drops may work. For severe cases, topical corticosteroids help, but you need to be closely monitored for cataracts, glaucoma, or infections of the cornea.

Prescribed medications in the form of eye drops are very effective in alleviating symptoms. Drops with antihistamines, mast cell stabilizers, or both have few side effects. Topical decongestants don't treat the underlying cause, but can decrease eye redness and relieve itching. They are often combined with antihistamines. Side effects may include blurred vision or some stinging.

OPHTHALMIC PREPARATIONS FOR ALLERGIC CONJUNCTIVITIS

Trade Name	Generic Name
Antihistamines	
Livostin	levocabastine hydrochloride

Topical antihistamines provide rapid relief for acute ocular symptoms, particularly itching. Oral antihistamines provide only partial relief.

Trade Name	Generic Name

Antihistamine Vasoconstrictor Combination

Naphcon-A	pheniramine and naphazoline
Opcon-A	"
OcuHist	"
Vasocon-A	antazoline, naphazoline

Naphcon-A and OcuHist can help stop itching. If you are at risk for glaucoma, however, don't use them.

Mast Cell Stabilizers

Crolom	cromolyn sodium
Alomide	lodoxamide tromethamine

Antihistamine/Mast Cell Stabilizers

Zaditor	ketotifen fumarate
Patanol	olopatadine hydrochloride

Nonsteroid Antiinflammatory Medications (NSAIDS)

Acular	ketorolac tromethamine

NSAIDS are excellent for the symptomatic relief of itching.

Corticosteroids

Dexamethasone

Fluorometholone

Fluorometholone acetate

Loteprednol etabanate (Alrex)

Prednisone acetate

Prednisolone sodium phosphate

USING EYE DROPS CORRECTLY

Eye drops can be difficult to use, and unless you do it properly, you won't get the full benefit of them. Whether you approach your eye from the top or side, you must tilt your head back. Once the drops are in you need to blink several times to spread the medicine around the upper eyelid area. Keep the drops in the fridge because they feel good when they are cool when used.

When administering multiple eye medications, wait 5 to 15 minutes before delivering the second medication to the same eye so you don't dilute it.

Avoid contaminating your eye dispenser from contact with your eye, eyelid, eyelashes, or finger. Wipe it so water doesn't get into the bottle, but don't worry too much. Drops contain an additive to stop bacteria from getting inside.

Pregnancy and Allergy Medications

If you are pregnant, your hormones are in a state of flux, and affect your entire body, including your immune system. In addition, your growing fetus is a foreign invader—according to your immune system—because half its genes come from the father. Important changes occur in the immune system during the pregnancy to prevent the rejection of the fetus. We don't yet know all the means by which the immune system adjusts and permits the baby to grow, but researchers have demonstrated the following changes, among others.

- Variable changes in the allergy antibody IgE
- Changes in the number of white blood cells (some increase, some decrease)
- Changes in the levels of chemical mediators of allergic reactions, including histamine

With these alterations in the immune system, you would expect dramatic effects on allergies in pregnant women. But this is not always the case. With some women allergies clear up during pregnancy, some get worse, and still others have no significant change.

Hormonal changes also affect the lining of your nasal passages. The result is a condition known as vasomotor rhinitis of pregnancy. This causes nasal congestion, which is usually most noticeable in the last four to five months. It affects about a third of pregnant women. A complication of rhinitis is sinusitis, which is about six times more common in pregnant women than nonpregnant women. This can happen whether or not you have allergies.

IN THE FIRST TRIMESTER

If you have bad enough seasonal allergies that you would be very uncomfortable without medications—and you are not already pregnant—you may want to try to plan your pregnancy so that the first trimester is not in the pollen season that brings on your symptoms. It is in these first three months that it is most important to take no medicines, or as few as possible, and only those that have been cleared as safe for use during pregnancy.

Because the fetus is so vulnerable during this first trimester, ask your doctor before taking medication during a time in which you might be trying to conceive. Find out whether the medicine poses any risk to a developing fetus.

Pharmaceutical companies won't test drugs in pregnant women because it's too expensive. They just label the drugs "don't use if you are pregnant." Drugs are rated based on long-term use with no side effects and placed in one of these categories:

A. No problems in animals studied, no problems in human studies

B. No problem in animals, but not tested in humans
C. No animal or human testing

Certain antihistamines may be safe to use, but only on your doctor's recommendation and with great caution. Chlorpheniramine and PBZ are considered the safest in pregnancy. The next choice would be diphenhydramine (Benadryl). Never take high doses of antihistamines, particularly near the end of pregnancy.

The only oral decongestant considered safe during pregnancy is pseudoephedrine, but check with your doctor, as it affects blood vessels.

The apparent safety of inhaled steroids in pregnant women with asthma suggests that the nasal forms of this type are safe to treat allergic rhinitis. Beclomethasone and Budesonide seem to be safe. Aim always for the lowest effective dose. One of the better medications in terms of safety and effectiveness in treating allergic rhinitis is a cromolyn in topical form (Nasalcrom for the nose and Crolom or Opticrom for the eyes). The drawback is that this medicine is strictly preventive and only lasts for about 6 hours.

Avoidance of allergens is especially important during pregnancy. If you can tough it out through pregnancy without using any medications, that may be the best course. But be guided by your obstetrician.

Once the baby is born, discuss medications with

your pediatrician, because almost all drugs go through breast milk.

PREGNANCY AND IMMUNOTHERAPY

If you have perennial rhinitis or severe seasonal rhinitis, and anticipate that you would like to become pregnant in a year or so, you might consider getting immunotherapy. If you are a good candidate for this type of treatment, it may be worthwhile to undertake it as a preventive, so that you do not feel the need for medication during pregnancy.

A large study of pregnant women has demonstrated the safety of immunotherapy during pregnancy. But it should be started well before pregnancy, not only so that you will have improved by the time you are pregnant, but also to avoid the chance of an adverse reaction to a shot. This is less likely once a maintenance dose is achieved. (See chapter 9.)

If you are already on immunotherapy, it appears safe to continue. The dose is never increased during pregnancy. An increased dose has the potential to cause a systemic reaction severe enough to require epinephrine, although it's unlikely. Epinephrine can induce the uterus to contract. There are no side effects of allergy shots per se.

Alternative Allergy Remedies
Are Not Proven

We all know what a powerful decongestant a bowl of chili or other spicy food can be. In fact, some people get a runny nose just leaning over a bowl of hot soup or tea. These basic and proven homey comforts are okay, but don't look for any effective allergy remedies in your health food store. There are many, many herbal remedies on the market for allergies, but none of them have been proven medically sound or even effective. Hundreds of extracts purported to help allergies so far remain unproven. And some have side effects. Many are plant-derived, and if you have allergies to plant pollens, it could be unwise to use plant remedies without scientific proof. Many pollens cross-react with other plants.

Herbal antihistamines such as stinging nettle (*Urtica dioica*) are available in freeze-dried extracts. Quercetin, a nutrient found in onions, has been said to inhibit allergic reactions and also is found in grapes, apples, tomatoes, and red wine. Herbal preparations are not considered drugs; hence they are not regulated by the FDA. Although some may help allergy symptoms, they are also potentially harmful.

ALLERGY CHECKLIST

✓ Medications prevent symptoms if you take them before the symptoms begin.

✓ Nasal steroid sprays are the most effective treatment for allergic rhinitis.

✓ Over-the-counter antihistamines make you sleepy, but the newer prescription drugs don't.

✓ Over-the-counter decongestant nasal sprays are addictive and can cause worse congestion.

✓ Many allergy drugs should not be used during pregnancy.

✓ If you can plan it, try for the first trimester of your pregnancy not to occur in the pollen season.

✓ Alternative allergy remedies are unproven.

9

IMMUNOTHERAPY: THE CLOSEST THING TO A CURE

Immunotherapy is the ideal medical treatment because it blocks the allergic reaction from happening. Therefore, you don't get symptoms and you don't need drugs. The downside is that it takes a commitment of several years and involves lots of effort and expense. For this reason, it's used for more severe allergies, when allergy symptoms are present most of the time, and when medical treatment doesn't help or produces side effects.

If you have mild allergy symptoms that can be controlled with avoidance and medication, then there's no reason for you to get allergy shots. On the other hand, if you are extremely allergic to both grass and ragweed pollens, you may experience intolerable symptoms during the entire summer and fall. Because you can't completely avoid these common airborne allergens, even with air-conditioning and medications, immunotherapy makes sense.

Allergy shots are not meant to be a lifetime endeavor, either, as one 90-year-old woman found out when she came to the office because her own allergist had died. When asked what she was allergic to, she couldn't remember, but she had been getting allergy shots for 60 years! This is an example of an unscrupulous allergist. After examination, some history, and allergy tests, it turned out this woman had no allergies. If she ever had any, they were long gone.

Allergy immunotherapy doesn't reprogram your immune system, but it puts the lid on it. As your body adapts to the small dose of allergen in the shots, it becomes tolerant and stops overreacting to the allergen. After years, the lid is no longer there, but because your immune system has been resting, it may continue to do so. Allergies tend to wax and wane. They may come back later, but be milder. The allergy shots are not curative, but it is unusual to have to repeat them.

How It Works

Immunotherapy is a series of injections to increase your body's tolerance to allergens. Doctors inject you with very small amounts of the allergens, gradually increasing the dose. It usually takes several months of weekly injections to get to the top "maintenance" dose. Once this is reached, the frequency of injections changes, usually to monthly. By this time or when you have finished your course of treatment, your symptoms are typically greatly reduced. Treatment continues for three to five years or longer if your allergies are severe.

The treatment with immunotherapy acts by multiple mechanisms. It does act like a vaccine in part. Part of the immune system overreacts and binds to the ragweed immediately so it doesn't get to IgE on the mast cell. Through your body's exposure to small, injected amounts of a particular allergen, in gradually increasing doses, your body builds up a tolerance to the allergen. This means that when you encounter these allergens in the future, you will have a reduced or very minor allergic response and fewer symptoms.

As you learned earlier, the basic allergy antibody is IgE, which is overproduced during an allergic reaction. If you are sensitive to ragweed, you'll have elevated levels of ragweed specific IgE. Some allergens in very small doses—as in the allergy shots—promote production of a blocking antibody, IgG, which interacts with the invading allergens. The IgG blocks the allergen from linking up with the IgE allergy antibody on your mast cells. If you are sensitive to ragweed and are receiving allergy shots of ragweed pollen extract, you will show elevated levels of the IgG blocking antibody. During the ragweed season, you will not have the sharply elevated levels of IgE antibody that one would expect.

Medical researchers have also discovered that during immunotherapy the body increases production of suppressor-T white blood cells. These white blood cells help to inhibit the production of IgE.

GRADUALLY BUILDING IMMUNITY

The best results come when the allergy shots are given year round. If you are being treated for an allergy to ragweed, the dose of ragweed allergen should not be increased during the ragweed pollination period. This applies to other pollens as well, and because you are inhaling it and getting it by injection, you have a higher chance of getting a reaction to the shot.

The first injection consists of a small amount of the least concentrated vaccine, or a diluted solution of the allergen vaccine. Each week, you get a slightly larger amount of the vaccine. The rate of increase depends on your degree of sensitivity. Usually you reach the top maintenance dose in four to six months. Then, you get the maintenance dose every month.

Sometimes the skin at the site of the injection becomes red, itchy, and swollen, forming a raised wheal. Rarely you may have a more severe reaction. Always stay in the doctor's office for at least 20 minutes after each shot to be sure there is no other reaction. Recent standardization of allergen extracts has improved results and reduced side effects considerably.

Once you begin immunotherapy, it's important to continue on a regular basis until the treatment ends. Otherwise, it won't be much help. In general, people receive treatments for three to five years. After that, sensitivity to a particular allergen is reduced, often for years following the end of treatment. This can mean you may be able to tolerate the outdoors during pollen seasons with fewer symptoms.

Are You a Candidate?

When all else fails and you are miserable with allergy symptoms most of the time, then it may be time to start a course of immunotherapy. It makes sense when moderate to severe allergy symptoms are triggered by allergens not easily avoided, such as pollens or molds, occur through most of the year, and medications don't work. People who get this treatment are usually allergic to pollens, molds, dust mites, cats and dogs, and stinging insect venoms.

Whether or not you want to take shots for these allergens might depend on how long the allergy season lasts where you live. Six weeks of moderate sniffling might be bearable, especially with the help of nasal steroids or nasal cromolyn, or antihistamines and decongestants. But if your symptoms last three months or more, or if they are very severe, then you might want to consider getting allergy shots. This would also be true if for whatever reason you cannot tolerate or do not like the allergy medicines available.

Anyone over the age of 5 can achieve success with allergy shots. After 60, allergy shots are less successful—but there are always some exceptions. Never rule this out.

If you take certain medications, particularly beta-blocker drugs for high blood pressure, angina, or other conditions, you may not be a candidate for immunotherapy. If you had an allergic reaction, it might be more severe with a higher complication from giving you the epinephrine needed to counteract the reaction.

You and your doctor must discuss whether you can successfully avoid the allergen.

WILL YOU PERSEVERE?

Whether or not you stick with the allergy shots for the duration depends on you. The Type A personality tends to stick it out. This is someone who is superorganized, compulsive, and never misses an appointment. On the opposite end of the spectrum is the teenager on the way to college. The dropout rate for average teens is 100 percent. Someone with a life-threatening allergy, however, is never a dropout.

The majority of patients do persevere with the shots as they realize it helps them. Others drop out because of the hassle of weekly shots.

The Christmas holidays present another phenomenon in the allergist's office. Between Thanksgiving and the New Year holiday, fewer patients come in for their shots. Then there is a big rush the first and second weeks in January. If your interval is greater than a month, however, you can lose ground.

WHICH ALLERGIES RESPOND BEST?

Immunotherapy is ultimately successful in up to 90 percent of people with seasonal allergic rhinitis and in 70 to 80 percent with perennial allergic rhinitis. Whether it works or not depends on several factors. First, the amount of allergen given as a maintenance dose has to be fairly high. We know what the top dose is for most allergens. Maintaining stability with the maximum dose is another variable.

Pollen. Grass pollen has been studied most widely, and immunotherapy usually lasts three years after the course of therapy.

Mold. Rhinitis from molds may be a more persistent problem, especially in humid climates. Immunotherapy for mold spore sensitivity does not always work as well as one would hope. The available extracts of mold allergens are not as pure and effective as the pollen extracts.

Dust mites. Year-round rhinitis caused by dust mite allergy is often exacerbated by seasonal sensitivity to one or more pollens. Such chronic rhinitis is a good choice for immunotherapy. Effective, pure dust mite allergen extract is available. There is evidence that children with dust mite allergy can be helped if they begin at a young age.

Cockroaches. This allergy does respond, because a standardized extract is available.

Cats and dogs. Sensitivity to animals can be lowered by immunotherapy, but the best approach is to avoid or reduce exposure. If that's not possible—perhaps you are a veterinarian—then immunotherapy is worth trying. A standardized cat antigen is available and effective. Up to now dog allergen extracts have been less than optimal, but improvements are on the way. Cat immunotherapy is given very frequently because no one gets rid of cats. It is definitely effective, but high doses have to be given.

Horse. The allergen extract is not as standardized as cat or dog, so most patients practice avoidance or use medications such as antihistamines before exposure.

WILL YOU REMAIN IMMUNE FOR
THE REST OF YOUR LIFE?

Immunotherapy is usually given for 3 to 5 years. Occasionally, people need a longer course. Once the shots are stopped, about one third of the people remain clear without further allergies. Some experience the return of some symptoms but remain much improved. Others will return to the original allergic state. This tendency to relapse is variable. Relapses may occur within a few months of stopping treatment or ten years later. But generally, if you are going to relapse, it is within three years of stopping therapy.

Some people hope that by taking allergy shots they will be able to avoid the kind of changes in their home environment suggested in chapter 4, but unfortunately that isn't so. Both measures are usually necessary.

You also need to be retested periodically when you are getting allergy shots. The allergy may settle down. Then, the maximum benefit has been achieved. After three years, get tested again. Find out if you are still allergic, or if you have developed new allergies.

THE COST

Allergy shots are expensive. They can cost up to $50 a shot, so a five-year course of therapy can cost $4,000. Most types of medical insurance cover most of the cost.

Until we produce the drugs that will prevent an allergic reaction, getting so-called allergy shots is the next best alternative. There's a great deal of new research in this field, and some time in the future we may be able to take a pill to change the reaction of the immune system.

New Treatments in the Works

There are multiple allergy drugs in various stages of development, and the future looks exciting indeed. An anti-IgE drug is nearing final stages of studies before approval by the FDA to bring it to market. Because of the competition among drug companies, we don't know details about all the other drugs that may be in the pipeline, but there are a large number of compounds being investigated.

We are on the cusp of new types of allergy treatment that may be available in the next 10 years. For the past 100 years, we've had pills to block symptoms. Then we had allergy shots, really the first attempt to manipulate the immune system. Now we have the next generation of medications to more effectively manipulate the immune system.

Now, with the biomolecular advances in medicine, instead of blocking symptoms, we hope to block the allergic reaction altogether. We are looking at places along the system where we can throw in wrenches. We learn more every day about the immune system. In fact, breakthroughs in AIDS research have helped all research on the immune system.

The anti-IgE antibody is a monoclonal antibody produced in mice. Scientists then substitute 95% of the mouse antibody with a human form so no one has an allergic reaction to it. Because it is very complicated to make, this drug will be very expensive, probably too expensive for routine allergy treatment. It will be marketed for severe asthma. Because it cannot be taken in pill form—the stomach enzymes would destroy it—it has to be given by injection. It must also be taken over a period of time. But for now, while it is still not a cure, this is a giant step and a potentially very helpful drug.

Immunology specialists are also researching ways to make current treatments—allergy shots and drugs—more effective. Many promising products have moved from the test tube into animal studies. The next stage is human studies, which can take several years. One goal is treatment that will direct the immune system away from producing allergies.

One approach to solving the problem of allergies is to find drugs that block—throw the wrench into—various stations on the road of allergic response in the immune system. Another is to stimulate the path that leads to fighting infections. This redirects the immune response away from allergy. Potentially this can be done in several ways: by blocking the chemicals that turn on the allergic response; by increasing the chemicals that turn off the response; or by blocking IgE. We can also try to block the action of specific parts of the system, such as eosinophil cells, which are involved in allergic reactions, or stopping cells from sticking to one another so they can't send response signals. So far, we can only block the histamine, a product of the allergic response. We are also working on improving the approaches we already have to make them better.

ALLERGY CHECKLIST

✓ Immunotherapy is used if you have a life-threatening allergy or if avoidance and medications don't work.

✓ Immunotherapy puts a temporary lid on the immune system response to allergens, but it doesn't cure allergies.

✓ Allergy shots help you to gradually build immunity to the allergen.

✓ Anyone from the age of five can get allergy shots.

✓ Treatment takes three to five years of monthly injections.

✓ Not all allergens respond to the treatment.

✓ You need retesting in the years following this therapy.

✓ Many new allergy treatments are on the horizon; some may end allergy as we know it.

✓ An anti-IgE drug (monoclonal antibody) is awaiting FDA approval and will be used for severe allergic asthma.

PART III

The Allergic Person's Survival Guide

10

WHEN YOU'RE ALLERGIC TO YOUR JOB

Ironically, people in the health care professions are among the most vulnerable to occupational allergies. The number one problem for this group is airborne latex particles. Laboratory animal allergy is not far behind. Allergy to mice and rats is a common problem for scientific researchers. In fact, one study showed that symptoms usually occur in the first year.

One woman was allergic to mice. Both she and her husband worked in laboratories with mice. They took the precaution of wearing protective clothing, but the wife noticed symptoms at night in bed. Her husband had mouse allergen in his hair. Once he showered before going to bed, the problem cleared up. One positive result of animal allergy is that it leads researchers to do more research on these allergies.

Veterinarians commonly become allergic and this may become a disability issue. The only animals they can get allergy shots for are cats or dogs—there's nothing for all other animals. One vet was doing research with rabbits and was bitten by a rabbit. His arm swelled up and he had an asthma attack.

What can you do when you become allergic to your job? You've been working with animals for years as a veterinarian but gradually you've begun sneezing and wheezing as soon as you walk into your office. You've become sensitized over the years and finally, the allergy has come bursting forth. This can happen to anyone: a park ranger develops an allergy to tree pollen; a horse trainer to hay or horses; a gardener to pollen; a nurse to latex gloves.

Workers in flour mills, bakeries, and cotton mills often develop occupational asthma from airborne mold or fibers. And while this book is not about asthma, this occupational risk usually begins with symptoms of allergic rhinitis: runny nose; sneezing; coughing; and runny, itchy eyes. These are clues that something more serious will develop unless you take steps to control it.

While OSHA (Occupational Safety and Health Administration) rules protect us from toxins on the job, they do not always protect us from allergens. One of the more serious and widespread occupational allergens we've seen in recent years is the airborne particles from latex.

Occupational Rhinitis and Asthma

While you may have improved the air in your home, you are probably not in control of the air in your workplace. You may be breathing in allergens like dust mites and mold because the central heating or cooling system is not functioning properly. Most so-called sick building syndrome is, in fact, just poorly ventilated circulating air. There have been more and more discoveries about modern "airtight" buildings and how their air filtering systems and furnishings fill the indoor air with allergens.

As you learned earlier, cat allergens are in many buildings even when there is no cat present. Colleagues at work who have pets can be contaminating the air without knowing it. About a third of the people in most working environments have symptoms that may be related to airborne allergens. The difficulty is in finding out what they are and what to do about it. Talk with others at work to find out if they have any symptoms. When enough people report symptoms that they believe are related to the job, then there may be ways to get help through the company or building management to correct the situation that may be due to ventilation or other systems in the building.

Now that smoking is banned in most workplaces, the threat of being irritated by smoke fumes is largely eliminated. However, if you work in a bar, where smoking is still allowed, you may have a problem.

If you are already allergic, then you are at greater risk of developing occupational asthma. This is also true if your family has a history of allergy. If you develop asthma while working at a job with airborne allergens or irritants, then you should get tested to find out if it is indeed an allergic form of asthma. A pattern of illness associated with your workplace is an indicator of such a diagnosis. You may be coughing or wheezing at work, have allergic rhinitis symptoms, then on weekends or at night the symptoms fade. This association is not always clear, however. You could have a late phase reaction after you leave work.

Some of the work hazards may be obvious, such as animal protein in veterinary offices or on farms. Bakers can develop allergies to the allergenic proteins in flour and grains.

Dock workers and granary workers are also exposed to mold. Farmers, too, breathe in bacteria and fungi in hay, straw, and grains. Working with wet baled hay or in a closed barn in winter can cause intense exposure.

In certain jobs airborne allergens cannot be avoided. These include the following:

- Nursery workers, gardeners, landscapers, and florists.

- Bakers.
- Brewers may be allergic to moldy malt used to make beer.
- Butchers and meat packers sometimes get asthma from inhaling the vapors of the polyvinyl plastic wrap they use to package the meat.
- Carpenters. Woodworkers and builders of furniture are exposed to wood dust and chemicals used to treat the wood. The dust of the Western red cedar is a well-documented cause of asthma. The substance that causes it is believed to be plicate acid.
- Food processors and cooks can develop allergic rhinitis from plant proteins and enzymes. Mushrooms, coffee beans, and cocoa beans are fairly potent allergens. Cheese is made with mold. Simply inhaling the vapors from a food you are allergic to can set off symptoms.

Airborne Latex Particles

You may not be anywhere near a pair of latex gloves, but because the allergen in latex becomes airborne when powdered gloves are used, you can have an allergic reaction by breathing nearby air. While the latex itself may cause a skin rash, it's the cornstarch used in the gloves that carries the latex particles into the air. The latex protein adheres to the powder, and as the gloves are snapped on and off, the latex-coated powder becomes airborne. It's the main occupational allergy for health care, and more important, there's no effective treatment except avoidance.

Entire rooms can become contaminated by latex particles lingering in the air and landing on people, equipment, and surfaces. As they are inhaled, they may cause allergic rhinitis and respiratory problems, such as asthma. These microscopic allergens find their way into mucous membranes in your nose, eyes, and mouth. Such areas are particularly susceptible to latex sensitization.

Natural rubber latex is a common trigger for producing allergies. Estimates put the incidence of latex sensitivity or allergy in the United States at between 1 and 6 percent—or as many as 16 million people. Although this is very high, the problem seems to have leveled off, and fewer new cases are being reported. This may be the result of better glove-manufacturing techniques, and the widespread use of powder-free gloves.

The problem is that latex is the best substance to stop the passage of viruses, for example, from an infected patient with hepatitis or HIV, to the health care worker. Synthetic latex, which does not cause allergy, is also very good but is more expensive. Originally gloves had to have powder inside. If not, they were impossible to get on and off. Newer manufacturing techniques have made powder-free gloves a reality.

THE ONSET OF SYMPTOMS

If you are sensitive, you could develop symptoms if you are around people who use powdered latex gloves—for example, your dentist. Although the amount of exposure needed to cause allergy symptoms is not known, exposure to latex protein allergen at even low levels can trigger reactions in some sensitized people.

Reactions usually begin within minutes of exposure to latex, but they can occur an hour or two later and can produce various symptoms. If you have direct contact with a glove, you may develop skin redness, hives, or itching. The skin rash may be the first sign of allergy, so if you see this, be sure to take precautions before you develop other symptoms. More severe symptoms involve respiratory symptoms such as runny nose, sneezing, itchy eyes, scratchy throat, and asthma. These result from inhaling latex particles. If someone is very allergic and has direct contact with latex, especially via the hands of a surgeon inside the body during an operation, that person may experience a life-threatening allergic reaction (anaphylaxis).

Many things you use in your job and even at home contain latex. Rubber that stretches is the kind to watch out for. Hard rubber is made differently so is usually not a problem. Symptoms of latex allergy can also occur after contact with condoms, balloons, rubber household gloves, stretch dental dams, or any other latex products, or after dental or other medical exams or procedures where the doctor has used latex.

ARE YOU AT RISK?

Repeated exposure to latex means you can develop a sensitivity, and this ongoing exposure can develop into allergy. In addition to high exposure, if you already have allergies you are at greater risk. Children with congenital defects such as spina bifida are also vulnerable. As many as 67 percent are allergic to latex because their need for frequent surgeries exposes them to latex gloves on their mucous membranes.

Most experts estimate that about 10 percent of health care workers now have allergy to latex. That's nearly a million people.

Workers in the following jobs with ongoing exposure to latex are at risk for developing the allergy:

- health care and related services
- housekeeping and food service
- fire, police, emergency response
- funeral homes

- house painters
- gardeners
- workers in factories where latex products are manufactured

HOW TO KNOW: DIAGNOSIS

If your nose runs, your eyes itch, or you are sneezing, coughing, or wheezing after exposure to latex, you should get tested to confirm the diagnosis. A complete medical history is the first step. At present there is no standardized allergy skin test to detect latex allergy. However, many physicians have made latex preparations for skin testing, which are helpful if positive. A positive reaction shows itching, swelling, or redness at the site. However, because of the rare risk of shock, these tests are performed only at a location where staff are experienced and equipped to handle severe reactions such as anaphylactic shock. The tests are not 100 percent reliable.

A blood test is also available to detect latex antibodies. Another approach includes a standardized glove-use test, which mimics the occupational exposure to latex.

AVOIDANCE IS THE ONLY EFFECTIVE TREATMENT

Because latex allergy has potential to be life threatening, you must be careful to avoid contact. Particular care is necessary if you need surgery.

Use latex-free versions of products in your home or job and alert your doctors and dentist that you need to be treated with latex-free equipment. While latex seems to be everywhere and is difficult to avoid entirely, it is becoming easier as health care facilities begin switching to latex substitutes or at least powder-free, low-protein latex products. Latex-free trays, examining and operating rooms, and dental and emergency equipment are becoming standard. Vinyl gloves are available, but are less effective at blocking viruses. Use of powder-free latex gloves is now the norm in most medical centers.

TIPS FROM NIOSH (NATIONAL INSTITUTE OF SAFETY AND HEALTH)

Here are some ways to avoid developing allergy to latex.

- Learn to recognize the symptoms.
- If you develop symptoms of allergy, avoid direct contact with latex until you can see a doctor experienced in treating latex allergy.
- Use only powder-free latex gloves.
- Use non-latex gloves for activities that are not likely to involve contact with infectious materials (food prep, routine housekeeping, maintenance, etc.).

- Avoid areas where you might inhale the powder from latex gloves worn by others.
- Don't use oil-based hand creams or lotions when wearing latex gloves. This can cause the gloves to deteriorate unless they have been shown to reduce latex-related problems and maintain glove barrier protection.
- Frequently change the ventilation filters and vacuum bags used in latex-contaminated areas.
- Frequently clean work areas contaminated with latex dust (upholstery, carpets, ventilation ducts, and plenums). See chapter 12 for cleaning tips.
- Tell your employer, your doctors, nurse, and dentists that you have latex allergy. They can use non-latex gloves and also be prepared to treat you.
- Wear a medical alert bracelet.

CROSS-REACTIONS WITH FOODS

Just as certain pollens cross-react with particular raw fruit and vegetables, latex cross-reacts with some foods. If you are allergic to latex you need to be on the alert for this. (See chapter 3 about OAS.)

The following foods may cross-react with latex:

- bananas
- avocado
- chestnut

- hazelnut
- melon
- tomato
- carrot
- celery
- papaya
- potato
- kiwi

The reaction occurs when the immune system recognizes an allergen in the food that is the same or very similar to one in latex. The first signs of this may be a feeling of itching in your mouth or a flush of your skin followed by hives. Other symptoms may include feeling light-headed or short of breath. Severe sneezing, stomach or uterine cramps, or vomiting and diarrhea are also symptoms. Very rarely, your blood pressure can drop and induce loss of consciousness.

For this reason, if you are allergic to latex, it's a good idea for you to be evaluated for sensitivity to these cross-reactive foods. If you notice any of these symptoms after eating or handling a particular food, call your doctor.

EMERGENCY TREATMENT

Immunotherapy is not currently available for this allergy, so the only thing you can do is avoid exposure. If you have a severe allergy, you should always carry an EpiPen. Ask your doctor about carrying this form of self-injectable epinephrine, which can be administered at the first sign of a severe allergic reaction. Epinephrine, a synthetic adrenaline, works rapidly to reverse the symptoms of anaphylaxis by relaxing smooth muscle tissue in the lungs, increasing blood pressure, combating hives and welts on the skin, and reducing the swelling of the mouth, throat, and face.

Side effects of epinephrine may include momentary high blood pressure or a fast heartbeat. Some doctors recommend antihistamines like diphenhydramine to lessen the symptoms of an allergic reaction to latex, but antihistamines should only be taken in addition to epinephrine for the treatment of anaphylaxis and should not be a substitute for it. Only epinephrine can halt the potentially deadly effects of anaphylaxis.

You should report all reactions to your doctor. If you have a severe latex allergy, wear a medical identification bracelet and carry a card in your wallet.

ALLERGY CHECKLIST

✓ Health care workers are the most vulnerable to occupational allergens.

✓ Airborne particles from latex are the number one cause of health care allergies.

✓ Medical laboratory workers who handle mice and other rodents develop allergies in large numbers.

✓ Veterinarians often become allergic to their patients.

✓ There is no treatment for severe latex allergy except avoidance, so you need to carry a self-injecting EpiPen with epinephrine in case of emergency.

11

HELPING YOUR CHILD COPE WITH ALLERGIES

Young children often have head colds, runny noses, and stuffy noses, so how do you know when a child's symptoms are caused by allergies? Allergic rhinitis is very common in childhood. When combined with the usual quota of head colds, this one-two punch can leave kids with runny noses for much of their young lives. The first suspicion that your child might have allergies: look for stuffy nose and congestion. Some kids' eyes have dark circles, so-called allergic shiners. Frequently there is a crease between the tip and bridge of the nose as a result of pushing up the snug of the nose in the "allergic salute," which is a vigorous wiping of the nose.

Allergic rhinitis usually does not appear before the age of three because it takes several years for this sensitivity to develop. However, children who have high exposure to allergens such as dust mites may develop allergies earlier and have year-round symptoms. The most typical pattern in this country is the appearance of allergy symptoms between the ages of three and ten, then getting worse for about three years before stabilizing.

All in the Family—or Not

If you or your spouse have allergies, then be suspicious that your child's symptoms are indeed caused by allergies. It has long been known that allergies tend to run in families. As mentioned earlier, your child has a 50 percent chance of developing allergies if one parent has them, and 66 percent chance if both are allergic.

You can't control the genetics but you can control the exposure. And remember that genetics alone won't bring on the allergies—it's genetics plus exposure. This gives you the option to take steps to avoid or delay the onset of allergies in your children.

Dust Mites

Even without having allergies yourself, your child is still at risk as an infant. Animal studies have shown that there is an increased risk of becoming allergic to certain substances in the air when an animal is exposed to them shortly after birth. Similarly, we've learned that kids who develop allergies to dust mites, which are often found in enormous quantities in many homes, have been linked to the amount of early exposure to dust mites. Taking steps now to aggressively control dust mites in your home may reduce the vulnerability of your children to this allergy.

YOUR CHILD'S BEDROOM

It's most productive to find out if your child is allergic to dust mites. It's an easy test. Even if a child is not allergic, but there is a strong family history of allergy, it may still be prudent to decrease exposure as much as possible to try to prevent the development of allergies.

It might be a good idea to provide a dust mite-free environment for children in high-risk families— where one or both parents have allergic rhinitis, asthma, or eczema. (See chapter 4 for ways to rid the house of allergens.) This includes using zippered, allergen-proof covers on pillows and mattresses and washing bedding in hot water every week. Even consider covering a crib mattress.

Indoor humidity should be kept below 50 percent to inhibit dust mite population growth. If you use a humidifier or vaporizer to treat your child's stuffy nose, keep the relative humidity below 50 percent (ideally at 40 percent). Even if you strip the room of upholstered furniture and carpets, your child is bound to have some potential mite havens. Kids love cuddly toys—meaning stuffed toys—that they hug and sleep with. And there's that security blanket that gets dragged around everywhere and then into the bed. These are all homes for dust mites. Buy terrycloth and polyester stuffed animals that can be washed in the hot water cycle and put into the dryer to force the dust mites out.

Avoid Having Pets

If there is a tendency toward allergies, it's best not to think about adding a dog, cat, or other furry pet to the family. Once they become part of the family, it's impossible to give them up. Development of allergies to animals in children is associated with the presence of furry animals in the children's homes at birth. (Mice also produce a potent allergen, and could also be in the home without anyone realizing it.)

Your child is quite likely to be exposed to pets through playmates and classmates. In fact, he or she may sit next to the cage of the class pet, usually a hamster or rabbit. Talk with your child and the teacher as well as your doctor if you believe this is creating a problem.

Additionally, cat allergen is so potent that many people can become sensitized to it even when there is no cat in the home. Studies in Sweden and New

Zealand revealed that children in classrooms with children who had cats at home were likely to develop allergic symptoms, too. There is more about this in chapter 6.

Working with Your Pediatrician and Allergist

Because it's often hard to tell if a child has allergies and not persistent colds or more serious problems, you need to discuss the possibility with your pediatrician. Certainly let the doctor know your own history of allergies, and any potential allergens that may be in your home or involved in your family's lifestyle.

Your pediatrician needs to evaluate the symptoms. If allergies are suspected, then he or she will refer you to an allergist for further testing and treatment. However, your pediatrician can do a simple blood test (a simple prick in the finger) to check your child's blood IgE to find out if it's high. this test can be done before the age of six.

With moderately severe symptoms, don't wait more than a few days to see a doctor. If the symptoms are intermittent or very mild, you can wait longer, but you should not let any discomfort drag on for months without a diagnosis and treatment plan.

Children with allergies need medical attention in order to do their best in school and sports and other activities.

MEDICATIONS AND CHILDREN

All children taking medicine should be carefully observed and any changes in symptoms or behavior reported to the doctor. Medicating a child with over-the-counter drugs can be risky, so don't do this without talking with your pediatrician. The treatment should be discussed with a doctor. When you are buying a drug, tell the pharmacist the age of your child and ask if there are any warnings about which you should be aware.

When giving antihistamines to children, the main concern is generally sedation, which may affect learning and school performance. Some kids, however, respond in an opposite manner. They get hyperactive instead of sedated. One study revealed that a learning impairment could be partially counteracted by treatment with Claritin but aggravated by treatment with Benadryl.

Most of the new antihistamines come in dosages considered safe for small children, but they can cause side effects that adults do not experience. After taking antihistamines, some children may experience nightmares, unusual jumpiness, nervousness, restlessness, or irritability. Keep in mind the side effects of drugs not only appear at much lower doses but may also be different from the reaction in adults.

Children with allergic rhinitis can be helped by cromolyn nasal sprays. These are available without prescription.

If your child has severe allergies, he or she may be able to be treated with immunotherapy after the age of five. This therapy is often very successful in children.

Children taking oral corticosteroids may also be at increased risk of infection, including a more serious course of chickenpox. For this reason, those thought likely to benefit from intranasal steroids should be considered for vaccination against the varicella virus, if they have not yet had chickenpox.

If the recommended treatment is with steroid sprays, this should be done under the supervision of your allergist.

Middle Ear Disease (Otitis Media)

One complication of allergic rhinitis that can be serious for children is middle ear disease (otitis media). It can also be aggravated by chronic exposure to some irritants, such as cigarette smoke.

Middle ear disease is caused by blockage of the Eustachian tube, which runs from the back of the throat to the ear. In children, the anatomy of the immature tube makes it more prone to infection, with material entering from the nose and throat—a very short distance away.

The Eustachian tube ventilates the middle ear cavity. If it is blocked the ensuing negative pressure can cause fluid to build up in the cavity. If bacteria get into the fluid, acute otitis media may result. Allergy symptoms create lots of mucus, and mucus contains bacteria that can easily get into the middle ear cavity.

One study found that 40 to 50 percent of children who had chronic otitis media with fluid in the ear also had allergic rhinitis. The allergy symptoms cause inflammation of the nasal passages as well as the nearby Eustachian tube. And if the Eustachian tube is inflamed it becomes hyper-responsive to allergens or stimulation by histamine. The tissue of the Eustachian tube also responds to both early and late stage allergic inflammatory reactions.

This can cause earache and perhaps buzzing noise in the ear. If your child pulls on his ear or is irritable or won't eat, these are signs that indicate a checkup is needed.

Be on the lookout for any diminished hearing, especially in a baby or toddler. A child's hearing is normally very acute, and if a child does not turn toward or otherwise react to sounds, then notify your doctor so it can be treated.

Otitis media affects 10 million children annually in the United States alone, most commonly before the age of four, primarily because of the immature anatomy of the tube.

It is the most common reason for surgery among kids and the most common cause of hearing loss. It may be difficult to diagnose because at a young age, the child may not be able to complain of pain, or may not have typical symptoms.

The Link to Asthma

If your child has allergic rhinitis he or she is also more likely to develop asthma. More than 70 percent of people with asthma also have nasal symptoms, and about 20 percent of those with allergic rhinitis develop asthma. Up to 50 percent of seasonal allergy sufferers experience bronchial hyperresponsiveness (irritated airways) during pollen season.

Generally, allergic rhinitis does not lead to asthma unless you are programmed to develop asthma, but if you are, it then depends on environment. Ninety percent of kids with asthma have allergies. Once you have the inherited tendency for asthma, infection can also trigger the disease. It has been said that genetics loads the gun, and the environment pulls the trigger.

College students who had been previously diagnosed with allergic rhinitis were followed over 23 years and were found to be three times more likely to be diagnosed with new asthma later than those who did not have allergic rhinitis. Although the association between allergic rhinitis and the development of asthma is well established, a cause-and-effect relationship remains uncertain. The exact mechanisms by which the two disorders may be related are also not defined. They share the same lining as parts of the respiratory system. Nasal congestion may also lead to increased inhalation of cold, dry air and allergens through the mouth, leading to asthmatic response.

Allergy shots reduce the risk of developing asthma in children with seasonal allergies, according to a study by European researchers in the February 2002 issue of the *Journal of Allergy and Clinical Immunology,* a scientific journal of the AAAAI.

In this study, 205 children, each with a history of allergy to birch and/or grass pollen, were randomly assigned to one of two groups—the immunotherapy group and the control group. All children were given an initial evaluation to determine the severity of their allergies and whether or not they had asthma. After this evaluation, the immunotherapy group began treatment of weekly injections for the pollen they were allergic to, followed by maintenance doses every six weeks for a total of three years. The control group received no treatment. All children were allowed to take medications to alleviate allergy and asthma symptoms.

Among the 151 children who did not have asthma before treatment, fewer children in the immunotherapy group developed asthma than in the control group.

In the therapy group, 24 percent developed asthma compared with 44 percent in the control group.

After three years of treatment, bronchial hyperre-sponsiveness scores improved in both groups, but the improvement was more significant in the immunotherapy group.

Immunotherapy is successful in up to 90 percent of patients with seasonal allergies. The therapy affects the natural course of allergies by altering a person's response to allergens by manipulating the immunologic response. Researchers theorized that if immunotherapy is able to improve symptoms in one portion of the airways (the nose), it also could give the same immunologic protection to another part (lungs), and that it could change the natural course of allergic disease by preventing the immunologic response to allergens.

Information That Children Can Use

The AAAAI produces a number of materials for children to help them understand allergies. A coloring book called *Doctor Al and the Sneeze and Wheeze Busters* draws children in to the story of the good guys like Buster and Annie Histamine and the bad guys like Igor von Pollen and Darth Mite.

A simple illustrated book called *All About Allergies* shows children with allergies interacting with their friends and others. There are also videos available.

Go Blow Your Nose, Robert is a paperback book written by Nancy Sander and illustrated by Jim

Brown. It's a humorous rhyming story for kids and parents that teaches how to stop allergy symptoms. It is available from the Allergy and Asthma Network Mothers of Asthmatics.

The American Association of Pediatrics has a book called *Guide to Your Child's Allergies and Asthma: Breathing Easy and Bringing Up Healthy, Active Children*. It is edited by Michael J. Welch, M.D., and was published by Villard in 2000.

When children have allergies, it's important that they don't get the impression they are invalids. The message they need is that they can lead normal lives. For example, a football coach who is willing to carry around inhalers for players with asthma, and who praises those players, goes a long way toward convincing youngsters they can lead active lives.

ALLERGY CHECKLIST

✓ If one or both parents have any allergies, children are likely to get them, too.

✓ Your child can be tested early for the IgE antibody to see if he or she is allergic.

✓ Because of a child's immature immune system, it is hard to tell if symptoms are from allergies or colds.

✓ Dust mites in your home can make your child more vulnerable to allergies.

✓ If you have a history of allergy, avoid getting furry pets for your children.

✓ Children can receive allergy immunotherapy by the age of 5.

✓ Allergic rhinitis can lead to middle ear disease in small children.

12

AIR MANAGEMENT 101: MAKING YOUR HOME ALLERGEN-FREE

Can your home be 100 percent allergy proof? Unless you live in the biosphere, it's unlikely, but you can come very close and reduce your vulnerability to symptoms. Most of us don't even think about what's in the air inside our homes unless we are suddenly overwhelmed by cooking odors or paint fumes. But if you have allergies, consider "air management" just as important to your household maintenance as taking out the garbage and regular cleaning. The potential effect on the air in your home is also something to consider before you buy carpeting, furnishings, or cleaning supplies, and before you plan any renovation.

Clarify Your Goal

It's not necessary for you to take all of these measures if you are not allergic to all possible allergens, but set a goal in accordance with your allergy symptoms. If you are allergic to pollen, you need a good air-conditioning system to filter out the pollen from outdoors. If you are allergic to dust mites, you need the air in your bedroom to be especially clean, and if you are allergic to mold you need to keep the air dry; so figure out what you need before you begin. Do you want to absorb allergy particles from inside the house from a cat or stop outdoor allergens from coming inside? Once your goal is clear, you can plan the changes you need.

Changing your indoor air environment may take some time, so begin by making a priority list, such as improving your air-conditioning system, the ventilation of all rooms in the house, and patching water leaks in damp areas. Progressive changes produce a less allergic environment that will be easier to clean and healthier for the whole family. The best reason of all to take such preventive steps is if you are genetically prone to allergies and have children who may develop allergies from exposure to airborne allergens.

A thorough and professional housecleaning and the use of exhaust fans and well-maintained air conditioners and dehumidifiers are the best allergen reducers.

Get Hip to HEPA

The HEPA filter (high efficiency particulate arresting) is the only filter that can screen out the tiny allergens that circulate in the air. These filters are used in heating and cooling systems, air purifiers, air conditioners, vacuum cleaners, and even face masks. HEPA has a triple filter and traps the smallest particles and gases.

It's important before you invest any money to understand the types of filters available and what they do—and do not do. There are many types of filters, but the most common are the plain thick filters—usually foam rubber—that trap large particles and are not so good with overall filtration. Another type is the electrostatic filter, that works by imparting a charge to particles in the air as they pass through the filter and then trapping the particles with an oppositely charged plate in the unit. Such a filter could be used in a central furnace or in room vents. Electrostatic filters have one drawback: they may produce ozone, which makes asthma worse.

A disposable 3M electrostatic microparticle air filter for a wall air conditioner unit is 20 times more effective than ordinary foam and slide-in mesh screen filters at capturing airborne microparticles such as smoke and dust. It is less effective than a HEPA filter for trapping allergy particles. A large sheet cut to size lasts about two months and costs $8.

Whether it is a central unit or a window unit, filters must be cleaned frequently, both for maximum efficiency and to prevent mold growth. However, many cannot be cleaned and need to be replaced frequently.

Questions to ask when buying filters:

- Most important is what size particle does it trap. You want a system to trap down to at least 5 microns—smaller than the dot at the end of this sentence. Allergen particles are usually this size and sometimes smaller. The smaller the particle size trapped, the better. Only HEPA filters trap it all.
- Does it give off ozone? If so, this is not good.
- Cost. Quite often cheap machines need very expensive filters that require frequent changing.

Central Heating and Cooling Systems

Allergy sufferers find radiant heat systems, such as electric heating and hot-water heating, are generally better for allergies than forced-air systems that blow allergens around. Some forced-air heating systems come with a humidifying element to counteract dryness. But this can be double trouble because mold may emerge from the humidifying element if humidity is greater than 50 percent. The systems should come with instructions for cleaning and the cleaning must be done on schedule. If you are allergic to mold and dust mites, keep the humidity low.

Particles can spread through the house through the ducts in a forced-air heating system. These particles can be captured and air quality improved by the addition of electrostatic filters in the central furnace and at points of entry on the room vent. These offer high filtration efficiency with low air-flow resistance. They need to be replaced every two months. And remember—they don't get all the allergens.

A disposable central furnace filter means you avoid the chore of washing a permanent filter. This filter can be replaced seasonally. The fibers are permanently charged to attract and retain microparticles. It lasts about three months and comes in a variety of sizes and thickness.

It is not clear that the filters available for home heating systems are fully effective. Ask for guaranteed specifications on the size of the particle that the filter will trap. Five microns or less is good.

Effective Use of Air Conditioners

An air conditioner is almost essential to filter summertime air if you are sensitive to pollen and other seasonal airborne allergens. Outdoor allergens such as pollen and mold spores come into the house when doors and windows are open. Air-conditioning is the best way to clean, recirculate, and dehumidify the air.

If you don't have central air-conditioning, then make your bedroom a priority. Before you buy a window unit, measure your bedroom so you buy the proper size air conditioner. It must have a capacity for a certain number of BTUs to efficiently dehumidify, filter, and cool the air. For example, if you have a 12 x 18 bedroom, you need a window air-conditioning unit of at least 8,000 BTUs. There are formulas for unit size needed for different size rooms. The salespeople usually can advise you.

Window Fans

If you are allergic to outdoor allergens it is best to keep the windows closed. But if you need fresh air, and you cannot install an air conditioner, an electrostatic air filter window fan may help filter out some particles. These have reversible fresh air/exhaust control. Side screens adjust to fit most windows. Be sure the side screens fit securely, so that outside air doesn't leak in around the unit. If fresh air is needed and the allergen is outside, they are okay.

Dehumidifiers

If you live in a low-lying and constantly damp area like cities around the Gulf of Mexico, the Northwest coast, or in thickly forested areas, you may need a good dehumidifying machine in your home. While it's impossible for these to control the humidity in the entire home, they can be effective in particular rooms and areas, such as the basement, where they are most needed. If you are allergic to mold, it is probably essential to have a dehumidifier. Refer to chapter 4 on controlling mold for more details on dehumidifiers.

Room Air Purifiers and Cleaners

Appliance stores like to push their air cleaners during allergy seasons and periods of high pollution. But most of these devices don't really help. And worse, people buy a unit much too small for the room they to clean and it is completely ineffective. Faulty filters and failure to clean them is another problem.

HEPA is proven excellent at cleaning a small bedroom, but the average person spends only eight hours there. The rest of the time you are breathing allergens elsewhere. Nevertheless, if you can afford it, it may bring you considerable relief while you are asleep. It depends on the allergen—if it's to a cat that sleeps in your bedroom, then absolutely it helps.

Some air filtration machines use electrostatic precipitators and ionizers to control dust. Electrostatic precipitators have been accused of producing ozone, but tests of filtration machines with charcoal prefilters show no apparent ozone problems. Ask the sales personnel about the differences between machines and whether they produce ozone.

Keep the Air Free of Irritants

If you are sensitive to strong, harsh odors as many allergic people are, you need to keep irritants out of the air in your home. Irritants in the air are not allergens, but if you have symptoms of allergic rhinitis, then irritants can aggravate your allergy symptoms, or your allergies can make you respond to the irritants. For example, some people sneeze or their eyes sting whenever they clean the windows with window cleaners that contain ammonia.

Many allergic people have nonallergic rhinitis, an overreaction to nonspecific irritants such as strong smells, especially these:

- ammonia
- cigarette smoke
- perfume
- paint
- scented candles
- room deodorizers
- natural gas or kerosene
- chemicals in new carpeting or padding
- insect repellents and pesticides
- exhaust fumes from large vehicles

Symptoms of both are similar, except when you are allergic you sneeze more and have itchy eyes. Therefore, it is helpful to keep the environment clean. Most people with allergies—while they are symptomatic—will have increased sensitivity to irritants. Keep your home well ventilated and the air circulating.

Housekeeping Hints for the Allergic

Weekly vacuuming (with ordinary vacuums) can help to remove dust mites from the carpet, but it also stirs them up and can cause more symptoms. Most vacuum cleaners leak, blowing allergens back into the air. Leakage may occur through poor connections of hosing and wands, from the dust collecting bag around the closing seam of the unit, and through the exhaust.

The process of vacuuming fills the air with dust disturbed by the flow of the exhaust and by the movement of furniture. The result is that, in the short run at least, you'll inhale more dust while vacuuming than if you just stayed in the dusty room.

- Pollen and dust mite allergens settle out of the air in a few minutes.
- Mold spores and animal allergens remain airborne much longer before settling.

THE HEPA VACUUM

A HEPA (high efficiency particulate arresting) filter added to a vacuum will retain particles at nearly 100 percent efficiency down to 0.3 microns and will reduce the amount of airborne allergens dispersed during vacuuming. This is the only way to prevent vacuum exhaust from getting to you. Most but not all of the vacuum cleaners with low emissions rely on HEPA fibers. These filters resemble a paper made with thin, pleated, glass fibers. They are also used in air cleaners and some heating systems.

Miele vacuums with a HEPA filter with their completely sealed system are best at containing dirt and allergens. A study reported in the *Journal of Allergy and Clinical Immunology* in 1998 tested several vacuum cleaners for their ability to remove cat allergen from the air. The investigators found that the Miele Air Clean Plus and the Miele White Pearl, with double vacuum bags, removed the most airborne cat allergen. Other vacuums with double bags did not do as well and still leaked significant amounts of allergen back into the air.

Miele vacuums also come with active HEPA filters that include a layer of specially activated charcoal granules to remove odors. These vacuums cost several hundred dollars, so before you buy one, make sure you know what it can do. You may also want to investigate if more current studies have been done. Usually, one or two filters come with the vacuum. The rest you buy. An active HEPA filter costs about $50.

SURFACE DUSTING

Dusting your furniture with a plain dry cloth spreads dust into the air. Use a damp or oiled cloth. More convenient, but more expensive, are the newer throwaway cleaning cloths now available. They pick us dust with an electrostatic charge, like a magnet. This prevents simply pushing the dust around and making it airborne. There are also mop covers that attract and hold dust. A damp mop is fine on most floors.

CLEANING SUPPLIES

Many companies sell liquid and powder cleaning products claiming to eliminate dust mites, mold, and animal allergens from carpets, mattresses, or furniture. Save your money. None of them work very well.

PROTECT YOURSELF WHILE CLEANING

The best way to avoid stirring up any allergens is to delegate this activity to others and leave the house while it is being cleaned. If you cannot, then wear a mask while cleaning your house. (See chapter 2 for information on the HEPA mask.) These are available through dealers that specialize in allergy products or at a hardware store. Even if you have good air-conditioning and ventilation and low humidity in your home, dusting and vacuuming may bother you somewhat. It's impossible to have a dust-free home, but you can come close.

ALLERGY CHECKLIST

✓ Depending upon your particular allergies, make a plan to keep your home as allergen-free as possible through proper heating, cooling, ventilation, and cleaning.

✓ Good air-conditioning will help keep pollen and mold out of your house.

✓ Only HEPA filters can screen allergens from the air.

✓ Room air purifiers generally clean only a small room.

✓ A dehumidifier can help remove mold from the air.

✓ Dusting and vacuuming creates more dust unless you use a HEPA filter in the vacuum and use a damp cloth to dust.

13

THE ALLERGIC PERSON'S GAZETTEER

Traveling in Reverse of the Pollen Seasons

Before you plan a vacation touring the olive groves of Tuscany, check the pollen season in Italy. And if the Mediterranean coast appeals to your wanderlust, there's a big bad weed that spews pollen almost year round. The good news, of course, is that you need to be exposed to certain allergens over the course of at least two seasons before they get to you. If it's your first trip, you may not be bothered, but your immune system is well aware of the allergens and is busy getting ready for the next exposure. So if you return at the same time next year, Gesundheit!

Allergies are a global phenomenon, but not all allergens inhabit the entire planet and not all at the same time. Australia and New Zealand have a relatively low level of pollens while the United States and Venezuela are high up on the pollen ladder.

Keep in mind that when traveling, the climate and the season of your destination will also dictate your specific allergen and irritant exposure. In tropical, damp climates, you may have increased exposure to allergens such as mites, airborne molds, and specific pollens. A businessman from India has severe dust mite allergy. As soon as he gets off the plane in Bombay, his symptoms overcome him. It doesn't matter what time of the year. He has one foot out of the plane and his nose runs and he sneezes. He is okay in Delhi, however. Now he takes his medications before he goes and his symptoms are blocked.

Mountains have trees; there are weeds in the desert. The only place entirely free of allergens is probably the Antarctic, where it is too cold for anything to grow. And you're not likely to get up close and personal with a polar bear to find out if you are allergic to those animals.

The Tourist Board of Iceland actually promotes its environment as "a sneeze-free Mecca" for people suffering form hay fever. Buildings are heated at a constant level with hot spring water, they say, and this, as well as fresh air from open windows, keeps the indoor allergen environment low. Also, there is no large industry polluting the air.

Nevertheless, at any point in time, you can find a window of opportunity to get away from your allergens. For example, if you travel on the East Coast, don't go to Virginia in April, or New York in May, or Maine in June if you want to avoid tree pollens.

Camping can be fun but can also increase your contact with outdoor pollen as well as your chances for encountering stinging insects. Avoid camping during high pollen seasons. Check the pollen season of trees in the area. When you understand the patterns of pollination, wind, and weather, you can plan ahead to get away when the area will be less potent for your allergies.

To avoid mold, try high and dry climates like the Rocky Mountain states. The Pacific Northwest and most of Europe is free of ragweed (or there is less of it).

It will help you to know a little about the rest of the world before you plan a trip. This is by no means a complete account of global allergies. Naturally, we know more about the developed world than we know about the developing countries.

If You Are Allergic to Tree Pollens

If you are allergic to birch tree pollen, avoid the northern European countries in the spring. April is the prime pollen season, but it is later in the colder climates of the Nordic countries. The entire nation of Finland, for example, is covered with birch forests. Remember this pollen cross-reacts with other trees and some fruit (refer back to chapter 2). In Japan, red cedar is a major potent allergen.

Olive trees are among the most profuse pollen

producers in the world. This evergreen is very hardy in the Mediterranean countries, but most noticeable in western Italy and Spain. If you have not encountered olive tree pollen before, you may be safe, but you may not be next time.

The spring flowers of the olive tree are small, white, and fragrant. They grow in short clusters called panicles. These little flowers produce so much pollen that allergy sufferers have demanded some relief. As a result, the more common varieties have been banned in several western counties of Italy.

Watch Out for the Parietaria Weed

Parietaria is to the Mediterranean what ragweed is the American Midwest. One of the most common causes of pollen symptoms in the coastal Mediterranean areas of Spain, Italy, France, and Croatia, is parietaria, a member of the nettle family. It can also be found in the southeastern United States, but is not a common cause of allergy here. In southern Europe, however, it is the most important allergic rhinitis-provoking plant around. It has a very long period of pollination and can reach peaks of production at the beginning of June. According to studies by the Split University Hospital and School of Medicine in Croatia, this weed causes long-lasting symptoms.

In Sicily and southern Italy, where the weed even grows on the walls of the towns, this pollen appears first at the beginning of February and persists until December. As a result people have year-round symptoms. It is responsible for 65 percent of the allergic rhinitis in Italy, but less in central and northern Italy. A survey revealed that 10 percent of the children in Naples were sensitive to the pollen, as were 30 percent of the adults. In Naples, 80 percent of the people allergic to pollen are allergic to the parietaria weed, according to the Split study. In Dubrovnik, the area south of Croatia, positive reactions to parietaria is 92 percent, but this number decreases as you head north.

The flowering season in southern Croatia is from March to November. Parietaria pollen appears first in the beginning of spring and persists throughout spring and summer. Then, a second but shorter wave of pollination occurs from the end of August to October.

This is such an aggressive allergen that it is difficult to treat its victims with immunotherapy, because they need such a high dose that severe side effects might occur.

OTHER WEEDS IN EUROPE

Until very recently, ragweed did not exist in Europe. It has been reported there now in Europe, specifically central France, Hungary, northern Italy, Switzerland, and Austria.

Even if you avoid ragweed, a more abundant pollen weed in central Europe is mugwort, which happens to cross-react with ragweed. Mugwort is another weed that produces pollen everywhere in Europe between July and September. The botanical name is *Artemesia vulgaris,* and it grows up to seven feet tall with small reddish-brown flowers and a woody stem. It cross-reacts with ragweed, dandelions, sunflowers, and all daisylike flowers. It also cross-reacts with celery.

A POLLEN OF INDIA

Parthenium, a relative of sagebrush, is one of the most common causes of allergy in India. In fact, 7 percent of the population of Bangalore are sensitive to it and develop allergic rhinitis. This potent allergen cross-reacts with ragweed, so if you're allergic to that, you may want to avoid the pollen season of parthenium.

A Guide for Avoiding Indoor Allergens

No matter what the climate, weather, or ozone level, you also need to consider your indoor environment and how it can affect your perennial allergies.

HOTELS FROM ALLERGY HELL

If you're tempted to stay at one of those quaint bed-and-breakfast places in Europe, especially in northern Europe, you should presume there will be heavy concentrations of dust mites in the beds.

Those pillows have cushioned a thousand different heads—heads that shed lots of skin for the skin-eating dust mites. There will be less air control in a B&B; they may not be air-conditioned and may not have a way of controlling humidity. These places can do you in and you may be better off in a hotel, which is usually less damp. The better hotels must live up to certain standards of cleanliness and air quality.

All hotels clean the rooms, but the staff is probably not using HEPA filters in the vacuums and most certainly not keeping the pillows hot-washed and hot-dried.

Hotels often contain large concentrations of dust mites and molds in carpeting, mattresses, and uphol-stered furniture that can worsen your allergy symp-toms. Irritant fumes from cleaning products may also cause problems.

While there are now pet-free smoke-free hotel rooms, there are rarely "allergy-free" rooms. But you owe it yourself to ask.

Here are some other ways to avoid allergens whether you are staying in a hotel or renting a cabin or cottage.

- If you are sensitive to molds, request a sunny, dry room away from areas near indoor pools.
- If you are allergic to any animals, inquire about the hotel's pet policy, and request a room that has been pet-free.

- If you are allergic to dust mites, bring your own zippered allergy covers for pillows and mattresses, or personal bedding—if you can.
- If staying in a cottage or cabin in a forest or near a beach, make sure to have it thoroughly cleaned and aired-out before you arrive. This can reduce dust mite and mold concentrations.
- Get an air-conditioned room.

VISITING FAMILY AND FRIENDS

Indoor environments, especially during the winter holidays, can be sources of potentially allergic hazards: wet leaves and smoke from logs for wood-burning stoves; mold from logs in the fireplace. Strongly scented potpourri, candles, or air fresheners may all trigger allergy or asthma symptoms. These are irritants, but added to your vulnerability to allergens, they make you even more miserable. Heating vents may also blow accumulated dust mites and molds.

Avoid staying in homes of friends who have pets. Even if the pet has moved out, the allergen remains in the air for months.

Always take your medications in advance of such visits.

ON THE ROAD

When traveling by car, bus, or train, potential irritants or allergens can include dust mites, indoor molds, pollens, and other substances. Mites and molds can lurk in the carpeting, upholstery, and ventilation systems of buses and cars.

Before beginning a lengthy auto trip, try turning on the air conditioner or heater and open the windows for at least 10 minutes before you get into the car. This will help remove dust mites and/or molds that may be in the system.

Outdoor allergens, such as pollens and molds, are also potential hazards, especially when traveling with open windows. If you have these allergies, close your windows and turn on the air-conditioning instead. To avoid excess air pollution when traveling by car, travel in the early morning or late evening, when the air quality is better and you can avoid heavy traffic.

WHEN YOU'RE AIRBORNE

Airborne allergens 30,000 feet up may seem like a stretch, but if you are in a plane, breathing in allergens from the cat parked in its carrier under your seat, you can be in for a miserable flight. The cat owner sitting behind you may also be spewing allergens into your air.

We have created the same kind of sealed environment in planes as we have in modern office buildings. Fresh air is added regularly, but old air is also recirculated. According to a poll by ABC News, most flyers believe the quality of airplane air is less than satisfactory. However, improving the air flow means using more fuel, so airlines may not consider the health of their allergic passengers a priority.

Some—but not all—airlines use HEPA filters in their air-flow systems. While ordinary filters may catch the actual fur or dander flying around from pets, they do not filter the microscopic allergens— which are the secretions from the animal. So if the cat in the box under your seat is busy grooming (licking) itself because it can't do anything else for a few hours, it is sending allergens out of the box and into your face. And these allergens are recirculating through the air-flow system.

Some airlines will allow as many as five pets on board without any prior permission. Most allow one or two and they need to have reservations. One or two airlines ban all pets from the cabin, so call and ask. You may find that a pet-free airline goes where you want to go.

Call the airline's customer relations department and ask about its onboard pet policy. Let them know that you are allergic and need to know if any animals will be on your flight. Here are some other ways you can try to avoid airborne allergens when you are air-borne.

- Book a flight that departs early in the day, when the plane is freshly cleaned and the filters may not be as full of contaminants. Also, you won't be as likely to get on a plane that had pets on it earlier.

- If you are planning a long flight, a filtered face mask may help you.
- Always bring your medications on board. Take preventive medications before you board.

ON A SHIP

While you are at sea, you may be breathing the most pollen-free air around, but there are other dangers lurking inside the ship, such as mold and dust mites. On most modern passenger ships, there is an air-conditioning system to control the temperature and humidity. However, not all ships maintain these systems in perfect order. And on a ship you need to consider the same things as in a hotel. Are the pillows and beds full of dust mites? Are mold and dust mites growing in the carpeting that is laid down on metal floors? And what about in the pool and exercise areas? There is generally a lot more dampness there.

When you make a cruise reservation, ask about the qualifications of the medical personnel and what kind of care is available. Find out if there is a doctor on board, so you can get treatment or medication if you need it. Also, ask if they have arrangements with hospitals along the route to get somebody off the ship quickly in a medical emergency.

Visit Your Doctor First

Before you travel, talk with your doctor about any potential allergy problems. Have a pre-trip checkup to make sure your allergy symptoms are not out of control. In some countries you will need inoculations before you can travel there. It is very important that you discuss this with your allergist first. Anything involving your immune system can affect your allergies. If your symptoms are severe, it's a good idea to talk with your allergist before you go. You need to discuss your medications, differences in time zones, and what to do in case of any emergency.

CARRY YOUR MEDICATIONS

Pack all your medications in your carry-on luggage in case your checked luggage is lost. Bring your prescription as well, for the worst-case scenario. Bring more than enough medications and store them in their original containers, which list instructions on how to take them and get refills. When you are flying abroad, the original container also identifies the medicines for customs officials so you don't get stopped at security checkpoints for smuggling drugs. If you have an EpiPen, make sure it has the pharmacy label attached, with your name on it. If not, you must carry a note from your doctor stating that you need to carry an EpiPen with you at all times.

If you cross several time zones, allow for time differences so that medication dosage schedules will remain constant.

ALLERGY SHOTS AWAY FROM HOME

Most maintenance levels of immunotherapy involve monthly injections. If you are traveling for more than two months, ask your doctor to help you to arrange for a way to continue your injections. It is important to continue this therapy. If traveling abroad with allergy extracts, make sure they are clearly labeled with your name exactly as it appears on your passport, and are refrigerated at all times.

Before you travel abroad, obtain the name of an allergist practicing in your destination area. Your own doctor may know, or you can call the American Academy of Allergy, Asthma, and Immunology for a referral: 1-800-822-2762.

If possible, it is better to achieve maintenance doses of allergy immunotherapy before you travel for an extended period. This way, you know what to expect and are not likely to have an adverse reaction from the shot. Your allergy shots should be administered following the recommended guidelines: having supervision by a physician for at least 20 minutes following the injection, and having injectable epinephrine available for treating adverse reactions.

Be sure you have travel medical insurance.

Get the Facts First

Before you plan your trip, check for potential allergens at your destination. One Web site is the International Association of Aerobiology at www.isao.bo.cnr.it/aerobiology. This is the International Portal on Aerobiology, which keeps pollen maps for Europe, showing where the pollen is highest and lowest. For the United States check www.aaaai.org.

To find out about immunizations that may be needed for some countries, visit the Center for Disease Control at www.cdc.gov.

ALLERGY CHECKLIST

✓ Travel in reverse of the pollen seasons.

✓ Olive trees in Italy are a major source of pollen.

✓ The parietaria weed in Mediterranean coastal areas is a major source of pollen all year long.

✓ You won't get symptoms for a new pollen until you visit an area more than once.

✓ Foreign pollens may cross-react with domestic pollens to which you are allergic.

✓ Quaint bed and breakfasts are more likely to contain dust mites and mold than hotels.

✓ Bring your own allergy-proof pillow cover.

✓ Check an international pollen Web site before you go.

✓ Talk with your doctor about medications before you go.

✓ Bring your original prescriptions so you can replace any lost medications.

✓ Bring medications in the original containers listing your name so you won't have problems at customs and security checkpoints.

EPILOGUE

Don't Let Chronic Allergies Interfere with Your Life

Allergies, like any other chronic disease, need to be managed and kept under control so they don't become so pervasive that you cannot function. In addition to following your allergy management program, it's important to stay healthy and avoid other illnesses. Maintain a good healthy lifestyle without smoking or using alcohol or drugs to excess. If you eat balanced and nutritional meals, drink lots of water, get enough rest and exercise, and deal with any illness—such as a cold—immediately, you can keep allergies under control. For example, if you often get colds, your allergies will hit you harder, too. Colds disrupt the lining of the nose so more allergy particles can now get one layer deeper and stimulate the allergy system. If your immune system is actively fighting infections, it may also overreact to a cat in the house. Chronic colds and upper respiratory diseases can make you more vulnerable to allergies. If your nose is always full of mucus, it's like Velcro to bacteria and viruses that enter the airways. This kind of benign neglect, it is now believed, can lead to a chronic state of inflammation that may contribute to more serious diseases in the airways.

Chronic allergies can lead to sinus infections, ear infections, and emotional depression and stress. Studies from the National Institutes of Health show that the relationships between allergic rhinitis and these diseases (as well as nasal polyposis and respiratory infections) are very strong—in both adults and children.

SINUSITIS

Colds are the most common cause of acute sinusitis, but if you have allergies—especially year-long chronic allergies—you may also be predisposed to develop sinusitis. Studies of people with acute sinusitis have identified allergy as a contributing factor in 25 to 30 percent of cases. Researchers have also reported an association between extensive sinus disease and allergy in 78 percent of the people with chronic sinusitis who were evaluated.

Allergies can trigger inflammation of the sinuses and nasal mucous linings. This inflammation prevents the sinus cavities from clearing out bacteria, and increases your chances of developing secondary bacterial sinusitis. Your doctor can prescribe appropriate medications to control your symptoms, and reduce your risk of developing an infection.

If you have sinus problems and allergies, it's even more important to avoid environmental irritants such as tobacco smoke and strong chemical odors, which may increase your symptoms. Although many symptoms are similar, sinusitis differs from allergic rhinitis, or nonallergic rhinitis. Rhinitis is an inflammation of the mucous membranes of the nose—not the sinuses.

The primary function of your sinuses is to warm, moisten, and filter the air in the nasal cavity. They also play a role in our ability to vocalize certain sounds.

Sinusitis, which is common in the winter, may last for months or years if it's not treated properly, and thus complicate the treatment of allergies. Cold weather and dry indoor heat both increase nasal congestion and block sinus drainage.

Sinusitis can affect the nose, and may be accompanied by profuse, thick, colored nasal drainage, bad-tasting postnasal drip, cough, head congestion, and headache. Symptoms may also include a plugged-up nose, a feeling of facial swelling, toothache, constant tiredness, and occasionally, a fever.

Acute sinusitis is often caused by a bacterial infection and usually develops as a complication five to ten days after the first symptoms of a viral respiratory infection such as a common cold. Chronic sinusitis caused by bacterial infections can become a chronic inflammatory disorder similar to asthma.

Structural problems in your nose, such as narrow drainage passages, tumors or polyps, or a deviated nasal septum, may be another cause of sinusitis, as they block normal sinus drainage. Stagnant mucus in the sinus is more likely to get infected. Surgery is sometimes needed to correct these problems. Many people with recurring or chronic sinusitis have more than one factor that predisposes them to infection. So, addressing only one factor may not be enough.

TREATMENT

Sinus infections generally require a combination of medications. In addition to prescribing an antibiotic when the cause is bacterial infection, your doctor may prescribe a medication to reduce blockage of your nose or control allergies. This will help keep the sinus passages open. This may be a decongestant, a mucus-thinning medicine, or a cortisone-like nasal spray. Antihistamines, cromolyn, and topical steroid nasal sprays help to control allergic inflammation.

Long-term treatment to control and reduce allergic symptoms can also help to prevent the development of sinusitis. Preventive use of low-dose antibiotics and sinus-drainage medications during times of increased susceptibility, such as winter, may also prevent sinusitis.

Several nondrug treatments are also helpful. This includes breathing in hot, moist air, applying hot packs, and washing the nasal cavities with salt water. In cases of obstructed sinus passages that may require surgery, your allergist will refer you to an otorhinolaryngologist, or an ear-nose-throat specialist (ENT).

Depression and Stress

If your nose is always running or you sneeze constantly, your nose gets red and puffy. It hurts from blowing and wiping. Your eyes tear. If you are a woman your makeup is always a mess. You carry around crumpled tissues and hankies. Uncontrolled allergy symptoms absolutely affect your emotions and sense of well-being. Therefore, they cause you stress. They can impair your quality of life, affect important life decisions such as where to live and work, whether or not you can have pets, knowing that your kids are likely to have allergies.

Never ignore your allergies, or accept them as your fate in life. For those who say, "Oh, well, it runs in the family, what can I do?"—you can do plenty, and it is by taking action that you will lift your spirits and not let allergies own you. Remember those F words for people who were living with allergy symptoms (foggy, full-headed, out of focus) most of their lives before coming to get treatment.

If you are congested all the time, your head is always full and you feel fuzzy, you don't feel good. You may not have energy. If you are prone to depression, you pay more attention to how bad you feel. Everyone's perception is different, of course. But if you have the blahs because of allergies, this may become your constant state of mind and body.

ONE LAST ALLERGY CHECKLIST

✓ Don't suffer with allergy symptoms as a fact of your life.

✓ Learn all you can about your allergies and how to manage them.

✓ Make a total plan of avoidance and treatment to manage living with allergies but without symptoms.

✓ Learn more about avoidance (the number one cure).

✓ Work with your allergist to improve your life.

✓ Medications have improved and work if you take them the right way.

✓ Immunotherapy is the closest thing to a cure and works if medication and avoidance cannot.

✓ Get allergy tested periodically.

✓ And remember, never date a cat owner.

GLOSSARY

Allergen immunotherapy (allergy vaccine therapy, allergy shots): a form of long-term therapy consisting of repeated administration of increasing doses of specific allergens to patients with IgE-mediated conditions to reduce disease severity from natural exposure to these allergens.

Allergen: the source of an allergy-producing substance such as pollen, mold spores, animal proteins, dust mites, foods, insect venoms, and drugs.

Allergic diseases: the clinical manifestations of adverse immune responses (including IgE responses), following repeated contact with allergens. Includes allergic rhinitis, allergic conjunctivitis, asthma, as well as food and drug allergies.

Allergy: a tendency to develop adverse immune reactions to normally innocuous substances (including IgE antibody responses to allergens).

Anaphylaxis: the most severe form of allergic reaction. It is a rapid, immune-mediated, systemic reaction to allergens. The reaction occurs rapidly and often dramatically, and is usually unanticipated. Signs and symptoms may include faintness, syncope, severe difficulty breathing, and throat closing. Symptoms generally start within 15 to 30 minutes from exposure to the allergen, occasionally begin after one hour, and rarely occur hours later. Anaphylaxis is always a medical emergency.

Antihistamines: drugs that inhibit allergy symptoms by blocking the actions of histamine at the H1 receptor. Older sedating antihistamines cause drowsiness and/or loss of concentration and may affect psychomotor performance. Nonsedating antihistamines don't usually penetrate into the central nervous system, so there are no sedative or psychomotor adverse effects.

Asthma: a chronic inflammatory disease of the airways characterized by airway obstruction, which is at least partially reversible with or without medication, and manifests as increased bronchial responsiveness to a variety of stimuli.

Atopic dermatitis: a chronic or recurrent inflammatory skin disease that usually begins in the first few years of life. It is often the initial clinical manifestation of an atopic predisposition. Affected children may develop later asthma and/or allergic rhinitis.

Atopy: the genetic tendency to develop the "classical" allergic diseases, namely, allergic rhinitis, asthma, and atopic dermatitis. Atopy is typically associated with a genetically determined capacity to mount IgE responses to common allergens, especially inhaled allergens and food allergens.

Basophils: cells of the immune system involved in the allergic response.

Conjunctivitis: a group of ocular disorders that result in inflammation of the conjunctiva. May be of allergic or nonallergic origin.

Contact dermatitis: refers to a broad range of reactions resulting from the direct contact of an allergen or irritant with the surface of the skin.

Corticosteroids, steroids, glucorticoids: medication with anti-inflammatory effects useful in many allergic conditions. Newer preparations for topical lung, nasal, and skin use minimize the risk of side effects.

Cromolyn sodium and nedocromil sodium: topical nonsteroid anti-inflammatory agents.

Dander: flaked-off skin from animals or humans. Secretions from animals adhere to their dander and fur and become airborne. The dander is not the allergen, but the secretions are. Dust mites feed on human dander.

Decongestants: drugs that relieve symptoms of nasal congestion or blockage by constricting the blood vessels in the nose.

Early-phase reaction: an immunological reaction that occurs within minutes of exposure of the allergen to the IgE antibody in sensitized individuals.

Eosinophils: blood cells of the immune system involved in the allergic response. They are partly responsible for the inflammation associated with allergy.

Hay Fever: common name for allergic rhinitis symptoms.

HEPA: "High Efficiency Particulate Arresting" filter used in heating and cooling systems, room air purifiers, vacuum cleaners, and face masks. The only filter that can adequately screen out tiny allergen particles from the air.

IgE: antibody of the immune system that is responsible for allergies.

Late-phase reaction: an immunological reaction that begins several hours after exposure to allergen and can last for 24 hours before subsiding. Inflammatory leukocytes (neutrophils, basophils, eosinophils) are involved but the late response is primarily mediated by eosinophils in atopic individuals. These cells release cytokines and chemokines during the response, which cause swelling and inflammation.

Latex allergy: an allergic response to the proteins in natural latex rubber or to the additives used in processing latex.

Mast cells: cells created in the bone marrow and located in the lining of the nose and lungs as well as other places. They contain histamine and are a major player in the allergic response in the immune system.

Mast cell stabilizer: a group of drugs that exhibit anti-inflammatory properties (cromolyn sodium, nedocromil sodium). The mechanism of action of these drugs remains uncertain.

Nonallergic (or irritant) reaction: reactions that do not involve the immune system. They can be important cofactors for aggravating allergic reactions.

Oral allergy syndrome: itching in the mouth associated with the ingestion of fresh fruits and vegetables that cross-react with certain pollens. It is not associated with life-threatening reactions.

Otitis media: an acute or chronic inflammation of the middle ear.

Prick/puncture test: used to confirm hypersensitivity to a wide variety of allergens, the most convenient and specific method for detecting IgE antibodies. A drop of allergen material is placed onto the skin, which is then pricked. If the patient is allergic, a hive develops at the site in 10 minutes.

Rhinitis: inflammation of the mucous membranes of the nose with symptoms of sneezing, itching, nasal discharge, and congestion. It can be allergic, nonallergic, or both. Seasonal allergic rhinitis is an IgE-mediated reaction of the nasal mucosa to one or more seasonal allergens. Perennial allergic rhinitis is an IgE-mediated reaction to allergens that show little or no seasonal variations. It is persistent, chronic, and generally less severe then seasonal allergies.

Rhinosinusitis: an inflammation of the paranasal sinuses that occurs with rhinitis. It rarely appears in the absence of nasal inflammation. It may be a complication of perennial allergic and nonallergic rhinitis.

APPENDIX A

Resources

American Academy of Allergy, Asthma & Immunology (AAAAI)
611 East Wells Street
Milwaukee, WI 53202
Phone: 414-272-6071
Fax: 414-272-6070
www.aaaai.org

AAAAI is the largest professional medical specialty association in the country, with over 5,700 members. Established in 1943, it represents allergists, clinical immunologists, and other physicians with an interest in allergies. The organization is dedicated to educating students and the public, promoting and stimulating research and encouraging union and cooperation among those in the field of allergy, asthma, and immunology.

American College of Allergy, Asthma & Immunology (ACAAI)
85 West Algonquin Road, Suite 550
Arlington Heights, IL 60005
Phone: 800-842-7777
Fax: 847-427-1294
www.acaai.org

Made up of 4,000 allergists/immunologists, ACAAI was created in 1942 to improve the quality of patient care in allergy and immunology through research, advocacy, and professional and public education.

Asthma and Allergy Foundation of America (AAFA)
1233 20th Street, N.W., Suite 402
Washington, D.C. 20036
Phone: 202-466-7643
Fax: 202-466-8940
www.aafa.org

AAFA was founded in 1953 to find a cure for asthma and to help control asthma and allergies through research, education programs, family support, and public and governmental advocacy.

Allergy and Asthma Network Mothers of Asthmatics, Inc. (AANMA)
2751 Prosperity Avenue, Suite 150
Fairfax, VA 22031
Phone: 703-641-9595
Fax: 703-573-7794
www.aanma.org

Since 1985, AAN-MA has worked to help families overcome and maintain control over asthma, allergies, and
related conditions through education.

American Academy of Pediatrics
141 Northwest Point Boulevard
Elk Grove Village, IL 60007-1098
Phone: 800-433-9016 or 847-228-5005
www.aap.org

American Association for Respiratory Care
11030 Ables Lane
Dallas, TX 75229
Phone: 972-243-2272
www.aarc.org

The American Lung Association
800-LUNG-USA (to find your nearest affiliate)
www.lungusa.org

**Healthy Kids: The Key to Basic Educational Planning
for Students with Chronic Health Conditions**
79 Elmore Street
Newton, MA 02459-1137
Phone: 617-965-9637
E-mail: erg-hk@juno.com

Immune Deficiency Foundation
25 W. Chesapeake Avenue, Suite 206
Towson, MD 21204
Phone: 800-296-4433
www.primaryimmune.org

National Heart, Lung and Blood Institute (National Asthma Education and Prevention)
P.O. Box 30105
Bethesda, MD 20824
Phone: 301-251-1222
www.nhlbi.nih.org

National Institute of Allergy and Infectious Diseases
Building 31, Room 7A-50
National Institutes of Health
Bethesda, MD 20892
Phone: 301-496-5717
www.niaid.nih.gov

U.S. Environmental Protection Agency
Indoor Environments Division
401 M Street, S.W. (6604J)
Washington, D.C. 20460
Phone: 202-233-9370

Indoor Air Quality Information Clearinghouse
Phone: 800-438-4318
www.epa.gov/iaq

Education for Latex Allergy Support Team & Information Coalition Inc. (ELASTIC)
196 Pheasant Run Road
West Chester, PA 19380
Phone: 610-436-4801
Fax: 610-436-1198
www.netcom.com/~ecbdmd/elastic.html

ELASTIC is dedicated to the promotion of increased latex allergy awareness and the prevention of future sensitizations through networking and education. It also offers information and support to those diagnosed with latex allergy, their families, and health care providers.

American Latex Allergy Association (ALERT)
P.O. Box 13930
Milwaukee, WI 53213-0930
Phone: 888-97-ALERT
Fax: 414-677-2808
www.execpc.com/~alert

ALERT provides educational materials and emotional support to people who suffer from latex allergy, as well as promoting latex allergy awareness, progressive policies in health care facilities and the workplace, and latex allergy research.

Foundation for Latex Allergy Research & Education (FLARE)
2501 Cherry Avenue, Suite 350
Long Beach, CA 90806
Phone: 562-997-7888
Fax: 562-997-8884
www.flare.org

FLARE educates health care providers and the public about latex allergy, promotes research to improve diagnosis and prevention, provides guidelines for hospitals and workers on latex allergy sensitivity and avoidance, and encourages government advocacy on latex issues.

APPENDIX B

Shopping Guide

Allergy Asthma Technology, Ltd.
8224 Lehigh Avenue
Morton Grove, IL 60053
www.allergyasthmatech.com

Allergy Control Products
96 Danbury Road
Ridgefield, CT 06877
Phone: 800-422-DUST
www.allergycontrol.com

Allergy Supply Company
P.O. Box 419
Fairfax Station, VA 22039
Phone: 703-323-1111

Aller/Guard, Inc.
Fleming Place Office Parkway
11121 South West Gate Blvd.
Topeka, KS 66604
Phone: 913-272-4486

www.Gazoontite.com

This is an online source of allergy products.

BOOKS

The Allergic Travelers Passport to Worry-Free Vacations by Dolores J. Sloan, 1992, Essential Science Publishers.

Ted Speed Press has published a book by Thomas Ogren called *Allergy-Free Gardening*.

INDEX

Printed in the United States
By Bookmasters